Medicine, Mythology and Spirituality

Recollecting the Past and Willing the Future

Ralph Twentyman
M.B., B.Chir., F.F. Hom.

Sophia Books

The information in this book is not intended to be taken as a replacement for medical advice. Any person with a condition requiring medical attention should consult a qualified medical practitioner or suitable therapist.

Sophia Books
Hillside House, The Square
Forest Row, RH18 5ES

www.rudolfsteinerpress.com

Published by Sophia Books 2004
An imprint of Rudolf Steiner Press

A catalogue record for this book is available from the British Library

ISBN 1 85584 182 7

Cover artwork by Anneli Twentyman; layout by Andrew Morgan
Typeset by DP Photosetting, Aylesbury, Bucks.
Printed and bound in Great Britain by Cromwell Press Ltd., Trowbridge, Wilts.

To Anneli

Contents

Preface

This small book, perhaps better described as an essay, is written after two decades of retirement from a life in active study and practice of medicine. A few words of orientation could help to explain how I came gradually to express such views, which are, one could say, fairly far removed from the current mainstream of medicine and from most alternative streams as well. It is not that I wish in any way to decry the great achievements of our times, which are absolutely necessary as the basis for a healthy development into the future. It is that I became aware, even from student days, of the overwhelming and universal nature of the crisis facing humanity and of the need to explore, as best one could, the very foundations, the paradigms on which our present civilization is so shakily erected. I was of course not alone in these heart searchings, however naïve they were.

Memories of my student days are vivid still, nearly 70 years later, and I well recall feeling particularly discouraged to discover that the basis for my future practice of medicine on living human beings was, bizarrely, to be the long months of dissecting corpses. My knowledge of Life and the living human organism was to be founded on a study of Death! Similarly, we were encouraged into an entirely inorganic and mechanistic view of human physiology by playing for many weeks with electrodes and a single dissected muscle and nerve of a frog. One day I noticed in *The Listener* a review of a book by Georg Groddeck, *Exploring the Unconscious*. I was struck by this review and went straight out to a bookshop where, lo and behold, this book faced me on display. After

buying it, I went to my room and read all night. It opened
perspectives of medicine and healing utterly new and revolutionary to me. Not long after this I was introduced to the
New Europe Group, an association of individuals from many
nations which aspired to hold back the threat of a second
World War by raising the cultural and spiritual level of contemporary debate. Among their circles I was privileged to
meet many significant men and women, outstanding
amongst whom was Dimitrije Mitrinovic, the founder of the
Group and a leading literary figure in Serbia. Through him I
received friendship and guidance in both personal and
world issues of historical and evolutionary character. He also
introduced me to the work of the Austrian philosopher and
scientist Rudolf Steiner and I met many of the members of
the Anthroposophical Society which Steiner founded. I was
21 then and the meeting with Mitrinovic was the most significant event in my life.

Two years after qualifying as a doctor I found myself in the
RAF medical service and then medical specialist (prematurely) in the RAF Hospital at Habbaniya in Iraq. It was a
valuable experience with, in addition, opportunity to
encounter numerous tropical diseases amongst the large
polyethnic population who were looking after the material
comforts of the RAF. However, after release from war service,
I was faced with the question of how to fit my career into the
developing National Health Service in Britain. I had already
realized the importance for the future of reintegrating the
Psyche and Soma, now so divided, and Groddeck's work still
inspired me. Before the war I had met many European psy-
chiatrists and also some homoeopathic physicians who pursued a psychosomatic approach. I enquired at the Royal
London Homoeopathic Hospital about courses and duly

enrolled, trained and qualified in this discipline and was appointed to the staff of the Hospital in 1948.

Homoeopathy originated at the beginning of the nineteenth century, at the same time as the School of Naturphilosophie flourished and as Goethe was establishing his way of 'Science and Seeing'. By the twentieth century homoeopathy was in a backwater, out of touch with current ways of thinking which were becoming ever more reductionist and materialistic. It became clear to me that for its long-term fruitful growth homoeopathy would have to find a link with an evolution of the kind of thinking which had appeared earlier in the Romantic movement, and in English literature with the works of Coleridge and others.

At this point, through the New Europe Group and its development as The New Atlantis Initiative, I was fortunate to meet Karl König, founder of the now famous Camphill Movement. He introduced me to anthroposophical medical work and particularly to the work on cancer and Iscador (mistletoe) therapy. It seemed to me then, and has continued to do so, that Steiner's most comprehensive work and method could offer the basis for a fruitful and healthy development of a medicine which was not founded on lifeless, mechanistic theories. Later, Owen Barfield was to write of anthroposophy as *Romanticism Comes of Age.*

Any radical new development, such as Steiner's (which he also called spiritual science), coming at moments of universal crisis and change of consciousness, must have been prepared over a long time. There were many men who caught glimpses of what was needed but, mostly, they are forgotten. Some few of these came to my attention and are on my bookshelves and have become almost friends. In the bibliography at the end of this book I have only included titles from my shelves, as this is meant to be a personal offering and not an academic exercise. The works of Steiner are, of course, far more extensive than those I have chosen to include.

In writing this book I have been constantly encouraged and goaded on by my wife Anneli and in the editing and preparing it for publication I have received most sympathetic and skilful help from Ann Druitt. To both and to the many encouraging and inspiring friends and teachers over my lifetime, my heartfelt thanks.

1. Order and Disorder

Anyone who has had the luck to watch, night after night and month after month, in the desert nights, the great star-studded dome of heaven move majestically across the skies will grasp how this revelation became for our ancestors the very origin and ruler of our earthly life and world. One can then more easily accept the recent discoveries in Egypt of the determination of the geographical positions of the pyramids and Nile from their correspondences in the heavens. A great star wisdom had arisen in Egypt and Babylonia in the cradle of our civilization and the heavens were the script in which were written the deeds of the gods. A last echo of this is to be found in Shakespeare with Ulysses' famous speech on order:

> The heavens themselves, the planets and this centre,
> Observe degree, priority and place,
> Insisture, course, proportion, season, form,
> Office and custom, in all line of order...
> But when the planets
> In evil mixture to disorder wander,
> What plagues and what portents, what mutiny,
> What raging of the seas, shaking of earth,
> Commotion in the winds! Frights, changes, horrors,
> Divert and crack, rend and deracinate
> The unity and married calm of states
> Quite from their fixture!
>
> *Troilus and Cressida* (Act 1, Scene iii)

In contrast, Lorenzo's speech in *The Merchant of Venice* (Act 5, Scene i):

Sit, Jessica. Look how the floor of heaven
Is thick inlaid with patines of bright gold;
There's not the smallest orb which thou behold'st
But in his motion like an angel sings,
Still quiring to the young-ey'd cherubins;
Such harmony is in immortal souls,
But whilst this muddy vesture of decay
Doth grossly close it in, we cannot hear it...

Tempest and music are Shakespeare's images for disorder and disease on the one hand and, on the other, harmony and health. Both are written in the script of heaven and both are in the will of the gods. For Shakespeare, meaning and intent are expressed in war and disease as well as in peace and health.

Earlier even than star wisdom, and the sense of heavenly beings behind or within those stars, was the sense for a multitude of entities in natural forces, for ancestral spirits and so on, which could curse or bless and which needed to be offered certain thoughts, feelings and rituals. Many traces of such a time survive in indigenous medicine worldwide, and Professor Ellenberger has shown in his book *The Discovery of the Unconscious* how such themes manifest even today in some of the most sophisticated psychological concepts and practices. Can we modern people find order, meaning and intent in such things, or is there at least a path to finding it?

The idea of 'order' must surely belong to organism. In past centuries the heavens were still conceived as a living organism populated by divine beings who revealed themselves in the heavenly script of sun, moon, planets and zodiac. Nowadays there are so many areas in which we are losing (or have indeed already lost) the very idea of *organism* which under the impact of molecular biology is being reduced to lifeless *mechanism*. It was not long ago that Agnes Arber, FRS, the foremost plant morphologist of her time, criticised modern biology for eliminating, of the four causes of Aristotle, all but the material cause. How can we most simply express these four causes? A house, for instance, only comes into existence if these four causes cooperate. Firstly there must be the man who orders the house so that he will be able to live in it: the *final* cause. Secondly there must be the plan, the architect's design: the *formal* cause. Then there must be the builders, whose strength and skill can build it: the *efficient* cause. Finally there must be the bricks, wood, mortar and cement etc.: the *material* cause. Ancient Chinese wisdom points out most pertinently that we *live* not in the walls and roofs of the houses, but in the empty spaces between them. We need to look elsewhere than the material or the mechanism to discover the reality of life.

The supreme example of organism accessible to us in this world is the human organism. Whereas animals have specialized in particular adaptations, the human organism has retained a certain omnipotentiality and has, of all the animals, remained nearest to the foetal form. In it we find the greatest polarities there contained in balance and harmony.

The notion of balance and disbalance appeared in the Greek depiction of the world constituted from four elements, fire, air, water, earth, to which was added a fifth—the ether. I think it would be a mistake to regard these elements as yet sufficiently densified to be perceptible to our senses. In the gradual densification from purely ideal, spiritual forms to our crude, sense-perceptible matter, these four elements were grasped as qualitative states. We may note that it was only in the seventeenth century that Van Helmont first described what we today call gas. For the Greeks, air was less material than our gas, and perhaps Ernst Lehrs in his book *Man or Matter* was right in suspecting that gas itself, and not only our perception of it, did in fact manifest later. To come nearer to the Greek idea we must approach this double polarity of fire and water, of air and earth in a qualitative manner rather than the quantitative measurement of modern science. It is characterized by the different combinations of the qualities hot and cold with wet and dry. What do these signify? Hot signified expansion, and cold contraction. We can experience this polarity in our feelings as well as observing it in, for instance, the mercury in a thermometer. How can we experience the quality of dry and of wet? We all know the difference between hard and soft water: soft water wets us almost without soap, whereas hard water needs a lot of soap to really moisten anything. We can also describe someone's character and soul as being dry, as in 'dry humour', or as wet, signifying that they do not stand up for themselves but combine with and give in to others. So fire is characterized as hot and dry against water as cold and wet. Air is hot and wet and rock, the essentially earth element, is cold and dry. In this way, we come nearer to what all this meant for the Greeks. Medically, this system of the four elements became interiorized as the four 'humours' on which was based the system of the four temperaments—the choleric, the sanguine, the phlegmatic and the melancholic. The choleric was the expression of the fiery yellow bile; the sanguine of the airy humour, of the air carried by the blood in the arteries; the phlegmatic of the watery, mucus processes; and the melancholic, as its name shows, of the heavy, dark black bile. Health was the balance of these four humours; disease was their disbalance or dyscrazia.

Side by side with this doctrine of the four humours was another way of looking at illness. In those days Nature was still experienced as a divine goddess, wise and loving; she had not yet become the exsanguinated mechanism of modern science. The symptoms arising in disease were recognized as Nature's healing efforts. The diarrhoea of various food poisonings, and so on, was regarded as her efforts to heal and should not be opposed but supported. Likewise, fever was the expression of her attempt to cook the foreign invader and absorb it. The fever should be understood as an activity of this natural healing force, or *Vis medicatrix naturae*, as it came to be known.

There was also in Greece yet another stream of healing—the temple, ritual healing. At Epidauros, and at many other sites, we can still wonder at the majesty and beauty of these sanctuaries. Sufferers came to these ritual sites and were directed by the priest physicians through moral and artistic disciplines. Only when judged sufficiently prepared and purified were they conducted at night to the Abaton, a special sleeping chamber. There in dream or vision they beheld Asclepius, one of the gods of healing, with his daughters Hygeia and Panakeia accompanied by snakes and dogs. Healing indications were given and snake or dog might lick the ailing part. On waking the sufferer could communicate to the priests the indications. In earlier times, in Egypt and in various subterranean sites in Greece, these rituals were more terrifying and were to some degree actual initiations into the underworld. There were upper gods that were approached through experiences in the world of Nature, and lower gods approached through plunging into the depths of the soul, the unconscious hidden realm where, if unprepared and unpurified, the soul could meet terrifying demons.

In this context we have to reckon with a moral element, an imbalance in the soul, involved in disease and healing. In the book of Genesis the origin of death and disease is linked with the temptation and fall of Eve and Adam. This 'fall' was described by Rudolf Steiner in his book *An Outline of Esoteric Science* as a descent into a deeper experience of matter. According to Steiner, mankind was anyway evolving into a more material existence but the spiritual being that is depicted in the story as a serpent brought this descent about prematurely, and hence also too deeply, with a consequent disordering of the human constitution. This is felt as sin, though only through this sin did consciousness of good and evil awake in the human soul. Disease has thus become linked with the idea of punishment and many people affected by illness ask the question 'Why did this happen to me?' The need for help in such problems led the sufferer in times past to the priest for confession, repentance and absolution. Today increasingly it leads to psychiatrist and counsellor. It will be the task of our future history and evolution to develop the radical metaphysical healing of the human race.

Two further ideas follow from these considerations. Firstly, disease is a disorder in space: a process that is right in one place in the organism becomes disease if it arises in some other place. Secondly, disease can be a disorder in time, when some development occurs too early or when an opportunity is missed and the development does not come about at the right time.

> There is a tide in the affairs of men
> Which, taken at the flood, leads on to fortune;
> Omitted, all the voyage of their life
> Is bound in shallows and in miseries,

On such a full sea are we now afloat,
And we must take the current when it serves,
Or lose our ventures.

Julius Caesar (Act IV, Scene iii)

Time and space create their own frontiers, so let us now look at the many frontiers dividing the separate realms of our experience of life.

2. Crossing Frontiers

We pass a major frontier at the moment of falling asleep and another, somewhat akin, at death. The idea of death has only gradually assumed a fearful and melancholy aspect, for in very ancient times, when people still felt near to a spiritual world and recognized it as a world from which they had come, death was felt more as a metamorphosis than as an end. In Greek times things began to change, and to die meant to enter the underworld, or Hades, and the frontier to Hades was the River Styx. All experiences beyond such a frontier pass into the realm of forgetfulness from which they can only be retrieved by 'remembering'. At this point in history death assumed a fearful aspect and the memory of pre-natal existence began to fade. Plato 'remembers' in the myth of Er the journey of the soul through the other world and its reincarnation into a new earth life. But later, Aristotle denied the pre-existence of the individual soul, which for him only came into existence at conception. The Catholic Church, in adopting the Aristotelian philosophy, adopted this great but not essentially Christian doctrine. It is obvious that these issues are of deep concern to medicine, so much of which is now concerned with problems of conception and of delaying or accelerating the coming of death. The confusion surrounding these issues leads to all the insoluble ethical problems facing medical practitioners today.

Bearing in mind that when we fall asleep we pass through a period of dreaming before entering the unconscious state (which, in his *Philosophy of the Unconscious,* Eduard von

Hartmann said might as well be called the superconscious), it is interesting that Steiner repeatedly reminds us that all human experience is carried on three levels of consciousness: only our thinking is truly awake, our feelings and emotions are in a dream world, and our motivation or will to action remains in the unconscious, or deep sleep state.

These thoughts of frontiers lead us to other motifs which concern the idea and reality of illness. Thoughts of poisoning and invasion are intimately involved in our attitudes to disease. Today, there is an almost universal fear of being poisoned by bacteria, viruses and other microscopic entities, or by chemical poisons produced by plant, animal, minerals and industry. In the past, at various times, there seems to have been a fear of being invaded by demons and other immaterial beings, whereas today we fear the invasion of our planet by extraterrestrials. Even our thoughts and our emotions can and frequently do poison us. We cannot weigh them, but that they have powerful effects is obvious to anyone. When we are ashamed we blush; when we are afraid we blanch. Our emotions may be immaterial but have material actions.

The venom clamours of a jealous woman
Poison more deadly than a mad dog's tooth.
Comedy of Errors (Act V, Scene i)

There is no need to get involved with UFOs to discover the reality of immaterial entities. What should be obvious is that poisonings or invasions imply the existence of distinct realms, separated by boundaries and frontiers from each other. We can see this historically in social fields. In India there were three main castes, Brahmins, Kshattryas and Vaishyas. Social health, harmony and stability required that these castes were kept pure, uncontaminated by each other and each with its distinct function. Crossing barriers between these castes resulted in social disorder and decay. No doubt the origin of such systems was to be found in heavenly spheres; the hierarchical organization of the Catholic Church, for instance, is to this day modelled on the heavenly Hierarchies. We now live in an age when distinctions of race, nation, class and even sex are being eroded. The old is breaking down and we have to create new order out of the chaos. Something similar goes on in the area of health.

It was Paracelsus (1493–1541) who emphasized that it was the question of dose which decided whether something acted, when introduced into the organism, as poison or as medicine or as nourishment. What in ordinary speech we call a poison is something which acts as poison even in a small amount, but 16 pints of water consumed at a go will bring about 'water intoxication'. The reality is that *anything* from outside an organism which continues to act *with its same nature* inside works as a poison! It must be overcome, digested, by the organism if it is not to work destructively. So snake venom taken by mouth is harmless: it is destroyed in the digestion and recreated in the organism as nourishment or medicine. But if a snake bites and injects its venom undigested directly into the blood circulation then it acts as a poison. Everything from outside, everything foreign to an organism acts destructively unless its own life is stripped from it through the process of being digested. A fundamental change is needed before such frontiers can be safely crossed. We can see this even on a social level in rituals of initiation and rites of passage. In most societies, when a child reaches adolescence and adulthood he or she must experience a leaving behind of the old life of innocence. A new life of adult responsibility is taken on and the young person now enters into communion with the men or women of the tribe or social group. Such 'rights of passage', seen as social 'digestion', correspond to the digestive and metabolic processes in physiology. A great wealth of such correspondences is already to be found in the works of Swedenborg, the great Swedish scientist-philosopher of the eighteenth century.

Let us look at some frontiers within the human organism. What was in ancient times *outside* us as social divisions, of caste for example, could be seen as interiorized within us as functions. Where shall we look for these? When we observe human anatomy, what strikes us at first is the division into distinct body cavities. There is the head with its cavity containing the brain. Then there is the chest, the thorax, containing the heart and lungs, divided by the great muscular dome of the diaphragm from the cavity of the abdomen which contains the stomach, intestines, liver and so on. When we are awake we mostly experience ourselves in our heads looking out or hearkening to the outside world, and thinking our thoughts. However, when we are living in our feelings and emotions we experience ourselves more in our middle realm, in a constant movement, largely rhythmic, which is closely bound up with our heartbeat and breathing. We are aware, but in a dreamlike way and, as in dreaming, it is difficult to say where we are in the ever-changing scenes of the drama. Finally, we must admit that, when in health, we are not conscious of what goes on in our abdomens; there, processes are conducted in a deep, unconscious state of sleep. The great dome of the diaphragm holds down, in an underworld, the immense activity proceeding in the abdominal organs. We are also unconscious of the magic by which our will to action brings about movement in the limbs. Our will is also in a sleep consciousness.

The individual relates to the world through thinking, through feelings and emotions, and through the will. Steiner showed that these are related to the nervous system and the rhythmic and metabolic functions respectively. Each of these functions extends throughout the whole organism but they are centred in the respective regions of head, heart and abdomen or as Shakespeare said, the liver, heart and head. There is, one can perhaps differentiate it, a fourth cavity, the pelvis, in which we find the reproductive organs in the woman, which are exteriorized in the man. When the head of the unborn baby engages in the mother's pelvis, one can see how it fits almost as a ball and socket joint. This fourth function we have located is concerned with the reproduction of the whole into a new whole.

Such are the frontiers of the physical organism based on the earthy, mineral skeleton. We must remember, however, that the living organism is at least 80 per cent fluid, not solid like the skeleton. This fluid body is further penetrated by air which, from the lungs, permeates the whole organism. It is penetrated also by warmth which works throughout in differentiated activity. Some organs are warmer, some cooler, some people have hot feet, others cold—and some have hot heads! We meet again the subtle frontiers and the interplay of these four elements earth, water, air and fire.

The dogmas held by natural science that only sense-perceptible phenomena are measurable and real, that all else is only subjective and fanciful has led to the present disbelief in the realities of soul and in spiritual realities. It is of course true that for our modern intellect, based on sense experience alone, the realms of soul and of spirit are inaccessible and therefore non-existent. Here is a crisis and a challenge. Is it possible for us to transform our knowledge and re-enter these inaccessible lands? It could be helpful to look at the origins of modern medicine.

3. Pathology Gets to the Point

Until the middle of the nineteenth century the old pathology of the four 'humours', developed from Greek times, still held a place. The last work on this basis was written by the great Viennese pathologist Karl Rokitansky (1804–78) who was a master of morbid anatomy. Up to this time, medical treatment had remained largely traditional, with the use of blood-letting and mainly herbal remedies, many dating back through the monasteries to Greek times. Surgery was still largely fostered by military experience and need. Then general anaesthesia was introduced using ether and chloroform, first of all in midwifery. (During the Middle Ages and Renaissance some use of opium and alcohol had been made.) This enabled far more leisurely, careful operations to be performed. Interestingly, it was through an early book of Sigmund Freud praising cocaine as an answer to human ills that his friend the eye specialist K. Koller developed local anaesthesia and opened the door to painless eye operations. In 1865 Lister began to introduce antisepsis into surgery and Semmelweiss brought hand-washing routines into the practice of midwifery and was severely persecuted for his pains! Concurrently with these advances, public hygiene concentrated on clean water and well-engineered drains and sewage disposal. At this time also there came about the discovery of bacteria and other micro-organisms. Largely thanks to Pasteur and Koch these entities were soon believed to be the causes of nearly all disease. War was declared on these universally occurring creatures and it was almost believed that disease could be abolished.

Surgery was able to advance, but not only because of the introduction of anaesthesia and antisepsis. Until the middle of the sixteenth century anatomy had made little progress beyond what the Greeks had achieved. Dissection of the human corpse had been practised in Alexandria for two hundred years; later, such animals as monkeys replaced human corpses. Distorted records of the Greek achievements, inadequately translated, were the only sources of human anatomy in the West until the Renaissance. A twentieth-century medical scholar, Charles Singer, has shown how it was actually the problems of illustrating three-dimensional organs and structures on two-dimensional paper that had to be solved before a useable textbook of anatomy could come about. Through the artistic study of perspective this was achieved.

It was the inspired activity of Andreas Vesalius (1514–64), a Dutch professor of anatomy in Padua, that produced the first real textbook of human anatomy, comprehensive and magnificently illustrated, based on his own careful dissections of corpses rather than on traditional sources. Medicine began to be based on structure, the structure of the corpse, and attention now became focused exclusively on the earthy, mineral element. Less and less was there a living experience of the watery or fluid, the airy and the warmth elements as constituents of the organism. In the eighteenth century the great Italian Morgagni (1682–1771) founded the modern science of pathology by careful observations of structural changes in the organs of persons dying of different diseases. Disease was identified with gross visible changes in different organs. Cavities were found in the lungs of patients dying of consumption, 'hobnails' in the livers of alcoholics dying of liver failure and so on.

At the end of the eighteenth century the French physician Bichat (1771–1802) had the use of microscopes. Noticing that some diseases were found at autopsy to manifest in structural changes in organs, he observed that the organs were a weaving together of a number of what he called membranes. He discriminated 21 different membranes, or tissues as we call them, and he related diseases to change in one or more of these tissues. The disease, though localized in a membrane, could therefore appear widely in different organs. In our time this idea is still useful. Rheumatoid arthritis, for instance, is regarded as a collagen disease. All the collagen tissues in the body can be affected, manifesting in varied symptoms, but commonly it is in and around the joints that we notice it most. So the seat of disease is still looked for in a structure, though now not so much in a three-dimensional organ as in a planar two-dimensional tissue. (Of course, the tissues are not strictly two-dimensional but they do seem to be interwoven in a planar fashion, reminding us that the typical organ of the plant, the leaf, is essentially planar.)

The great advance in medical science of the last four centuries has been based on concepts of the material world. It has been based on observations of the corpse, localizing disease in some organ or tissue and then, by the middle of the nineteenth century, in the cell. Rudolf Virchow (1821–1902) made use of the discovery of the cell to found cellular pathology. All diseases were now to be found in the cell. Organs were composed of tissues which were composed of cells, so pathology moved towards a pointwise conception. In this century, with electron microscopes and other highly developed technological inventions, we have seen this pointwise process move on. The seat of disease is now looked for in genes and other intracellular molecules. We have entered the realm of molecular biology.

As natural science moved inexorably into the sphere of medicine the human person has been progressively lost to sight. Disease is approached with mechanical concepts and the living person is reduced to a mere observer. The phenomenon of disease is disconnected from the inner harmony of the living, ensouled, human body. Riddles concerning the soul are insoluable and we have only the 'medicine of the corpse'. The soul has left the corpse.

Let us look back again to primitive times when the mythological consciousness prevailed, also in the practice of healing. A world of gods and goddesses was seen everywhere in nature as cause of the origin and continuing life of everything. The whole of creation was the expression of divine beings; everything was living. The earth was the earth mother under many different names and, impregnated by the sky god, she gave birth to all the creatures and mankind. In many myths the human race is formed out of clay or mud and water by the god. In Genesis Yahveh took dust of the earth and breathed into it and it became a living soul. The ancient mythological consciousness did not necessarily distinguish between air, which bears warmth so easily, and fire, and so Ovid told the story of Prometheus, the giver of fire, creating human beings from clay. The word human itself points to the earth, humus, and is in contrast to the Greek 'anthropos' the erect one. To be human is to have two natures, the earthly and the heavenly.

Long, long ages must have passed during which mankind lived in consciousness of a divine world of beings, perceived as real as we today perceive the sensory world around us, the world of colours, tones, smells, tastes and what we can touch.

The myths cannot seriously be relegated to a realm of mere fancy. They must be understood as the depiction of what was actually perceived in those days, in a more dreamlike consciousness, before the human being descended from a heavenly home down to the earth. Perception of that divine world faded over time and was lost. Today the modern mythologies arising out of psychoanalysis have pictured this state in the 'intrauterine bliss' of the unborn child. The mother's organism must be for the unborn child a divine being experienced in some consciousness analogous to the 'participation mystique' of the anthropologist Levy Bruhl. It is likely that these imaginative pictures of mythology are a better language for describing such early experiences than our current scientific jargon.

The mythological consciousness came to an end very quickly in Greece with the rise of the early Greek philosophers. The actual ideas with which they tried to understand the world have still much in common with the old myths, but the living beings, the gods and goddesses, have vanished. In *Riddles of Philosophy*, Steiner points to Pherykydes as the man in whom one can see the moment of transition between the experience of living pictures and the reaching through them with the exertion of thought to something that was felt to be yet more perfect and from which the pictures themselves were derived. Pherykydes, although mentioned by Hegel in his *Lectures on the History of Philosophy*, is largely unknown except as the legendary teacher of Pythagoras and Thales. In the two centuries following Thales, up to Plato and Aristotle, the birth of intellectual consciousness took place which, with its analytical, pointwise orientation, would have enormous implications for medicine. For Plato ideas were still living realities, the human soul went through reincarnation and

the individual pre-existed his birth and conception. For
Aristotle, the individual came into existence when, so to
speak, a drop of the universal became attached to an individual body at conception; at death all development ceased.
Plato considered the individual as a spiritual being who also
had a soul. Using Steiner's terminology, we might say that
Plato's individual had a higher and lower ego. With Aristotle
the human being has really come down to earth. Aristotle
invented the laws of logic and categories of thought, and
from this time onwards, as thinking became more abstract
and intellectual, men and women began to forget their
prenatal existence and instead used concepts, ideas freed
from artistic and imaginative overtones, to grasp the meaning of their existence. Wisdom began to be limited to
knowledge, concepts displaced vision.

At this time also, medicine became more emancipated
from mythological and temple dominance, and the figure of
Hippocrates stands as the legendary origin of this movement.
Greek medicine grasped illness in its individual symptoms
underlying which was a disharmony of the humours, as we
have mentioned, and such things as fever or diarrhoea were
seen as the expression of Nature's healing efforts. This
symptomatological view led to treatment by 'likes'. For
diarrhoea treatment a plant remedy, for instance *Veratrum
album* (white hellebore), which would itself cause diarrhoea,
was indicated to help and not hinder Nature's healing. But if
disbalance of the humours was perceived, treatment by
opposites was indicated. In the case of plethora (too much
blood) blood letting or application of leeches was the treatment. The idea of specific disease entities has only arisen in
modern times.

In the sixteenth century another crucial turning-point

occurred, though we can see its beginnings a century earlier. The alchemist Paracelsus, like Janus, looked both backwards and forwards. He had something of the old clairvoyant consciousness, but was also a precursor to the new chemistry. For an alchemist, substances were material and yet ensouled. The strict separation between matter extended in space on the one hand and a non-spatial, somewhat clairvoyant thinking on the other had not yet come about. The separation of chemistry and psychology came only after Paracelsus. The psychological side of alchemy has come to expression in the purely soul science of C.G. Jung. At the same time, a path led from Paracelsus through Van Helmont to modern biochemistry. In this way, psyche and soma, soul and body, were split. Descartes, who considered the body to be a machine and the soul merely a subjective, personal experience, is usually placed philosophically at the origin of this separation, which still plagues medical thinking. Today there is even a tendency to solve this civil war by eliminating the soul altogether, just as the spirit was eliminated progressively from Aristotle onwards.

4. Seeing the Picture

We have seen how pathology, the science of disease, progressed from the study of structural changes in organs to
those in tissues, to those in cells and then to the molecular
contents of cells. This way of viewing an organism as essentially a composition of cells is perhaps analogous to the trend
in chemistry and physics towards an atomistic tendency of
thought developed from the time of Democritus, inventor of
the idea of the atom, right up to the present day. It is really
only the physical body of the human being which our modern
mind can see. Aristotle himself could find no dividing line
between what was living and what was dead, between the
mineral and the living plant. Now if instead of looking for a
dividing line we actually see the characteristic features of
these two kingdoms, we shall be led away from a study of 'bits
and pieces' into the sphere of whole form. Characteristically,
a mineral substance is the same all through and it does not
matter to its structure whether we take a small or large piece.
Further, it is indifferent to time, unless we look into very long
geological periods and see, for instance, the chalk and
limestone mountains as the corpses of ancient living organisms. However, when we look at tissues or membranes as
Bichat called them, we observe similarities to the vegetable
kingdom whose characteristic feature is the planar leaf, which
is differentiated also in time. We could now go further and
look at the organs—heart, lung, liver, kidneys and so on—and
find comparisons with the animal kingdom. Then we discover
that we have moved from a realm of growth into that of
movement, or motion which would also include emotion.

The great, but overlooked, physician-biologist of the twentieth century, Hélan Jaworski, was able to indicate correspondences between various animal phyla and human organs. He had the picture that what is interiorized in man as an organ is exteriorized in nature as an animal. It is easy to see that our alimentary tract is an interiorized snake; the digestive juices can even become metamorphosed into snake venom. A bird is almost full of 'lungs' and their air sacs extend even into the bones. We could say that a bird is basically a lung served by other organs. We can discover that the female reproductive organs are exteriorized in molluscs, and recall how Aphrodite herself, the Greek goddess of love, came to shore at Paphos on a mollusc shell, as so beautifully painted by Botticelli. The cephalopods—the octopus for instance, with a muscular cavity containing the organs—and their eight arms, which in many varieties are flanged together in a funnel, are easy to see as uterus and vagina. In some species of cuttlefish the spermatophore on the end of a tentacle is carried to the female by the tentacle detaching itself and swimming free into her body cavity. For a long time, when it was found there in the body cavity it was mistaken for a parasitic worm. Jaworski also showed the worms as corresponding to the male reproductive organs. Out of this whole vision of Jaworski we are led to see the human not as a higher animal but as the synthesis of the whole animal kingdom. It is the trunk of the biological tree, not just the topmost twig, that is to be grasped as the embryogenesis or evolution of man, essentially human throughout its whole upward growth. As the different animal phyla were exteriorized as branches, so the corresponding organs were interiorly differentiated in the human body. How is it that Jaworski's ideas of man and animal meet with rejection by the scientific world?

The early nineteenth-century School of Naturphilosophie
had the work of Schelling as its philosophical base. Lorenz
Oken was a leading figure among these nature philosophers
and a contemporary of Goethe. Like Jaworski, Oken understood man as the synthesis of the animal kingdom. For him,
the animals were human organs become autonomous. From
this insight he went further and characterized animal
physiology as human pathology, showing how a process
that occurs healthily in the animal would be a disease process
if it went on in the same way in a man or a woman. A century
later, Steiner indicated that bees, for instance, whose life is
so dominated by sugar, can be characterized as healthy
diabetics!

In previous ages the human being was thought of as a
microcosm corresponding to the macrocosm. This way of
experiencing our cosmic dimension has vanished, as our
perception of spiritual realities faded. In its place, we can
gain the realization of the human being as not merely the
highest animal but the synthesis of the whole of Nature.
Although born from Nature, mankind is not *just* a part of
Nature. Another great scholar from the beginning of the
nineteenth century, Fabre d'Olivet, made a further contribution to this theme. For him, three realms become dis-
tinguishable: Nature is revealed as the realm of the finite and
of destiny, the spiritual world or Providence as the realm of
the infinite and, as the link between, man as the realm of the
indefinite. D'Olivet was able to interpret universal history as
the interplay of these three forces: Providence, destiny and
the will of man. The recognition of humanity as a distinctive
realm between Providence and destiny, between God and
Nature could be a helpful, even a decisive contribution. It
could give to science a proper functional role instead of its

present pretentious claim to be the sole and universal arbiter of reality. Humanity could reclaim its own distinctive kingdom between those of God and Nature and this kingdom should be the *kingdom of freedom*.

Modern medicine pursued its path and the sense for the livingness of Nature faded, but a last effort was made to hold on to this with doctrines and teachings of a vital force. Such a figure as Bichat, whom we have mentioned, was a vitalist and so were many leading scientific figures of the eighteenth and nineteenth centuries. But this vital force was conceived with the same abstract intellectualism as other forces such as gravitation, the electrical and magnetic forces, mechanical and chemical forces. No means of measuring such a hypothetical entity could be found and as organic and biochemistry began to flourish the vital force became itself unviable. The problem continued unsolved, of course, because the characteristic features of what we know as the three kingdoms of Nature (mineral, plant and animal) are all too obvious and divergent, whereas to a vision that accepts only atoms and molecules they are all three constituted from the same stuff. An important and helpful contribution was made by the eminent physicist Schrodinger who characterized the dead or mineral as the realm of the statistically probable, and life as the realm of the statistically improbable.

Our modern natural science originated from the fifteenth century onwards. Human consciousness was changing and, as Professor Butterfield of Cambridge showed, the conquest of Galileo's view over Aristotle's was not so much experimentally demonstrated as that more and more persons with Galileo's consciousness were born, and fewer with that similar to Aristotle. For Aristotle, light things rose and heavy things fell; for Galileo everything fell at the same speed.

Simple observations of, for instance, leaves falling, show Aristotle was right. Had Galileo gone, as we used to be told, to the top of the Tower of Pisa and dropped a feather and a coin over, then the feather would probably have blown away whilst the coin fell down. If we are then told that Galileo's view is true in a vacuum, we can only point out that in his day the vacuum tube had not been invented. In the course of centuries the human being had become obsessed with the earthly, the tangible. Materialism was the very foundation of a triumphant natural science whose ideal was the conquest of Nature. Measurement of experimental data now replaced full observation of phenomena.

Perhaps now is the time to consider Goethe and his way of seeing living beings. The great physicist Sir Arthur Eddington has characterized modern science as the view of a one-eyed colour-blind observer. He wrote:

> And so it seems to me that the first step in a broader revelation to man must be the awakening of image-building in connection with the higher faculties of his nature, that there are no longer blind alleys but open out into a spiritual world—a world partly of illusion no doubt, but in which he lives no less than in the world, also of illusion, revealed by the senses.

As the philospher-historian H.S. Chamberlain beautifully brought out in his chapter on Goethe in his work on Immanuel Kant, it was just in the gift of vision that Goethe's genius excelled; his was the vision of a two-eyed, fully colour-sensitive genius. His perceptions gave rise to thinking, living ideas. His perceptions were full of all the qualities of all the senses, whereas science has made the sense of touch pre-eminent and reduced colour, for instance, to vibrations or particles, photons, before it can apply mathematics to them. For modern science the truth of thinking is to be found only in mathematics. However, we find that Goethe, in his optical studies over many decades, used his actual *observation* of colour, especially with regard to the accompanying soul experience, the after-image and coloured shadow and so on. Henri Bortoft has emphasized how Galileo and Copernicus introduced modern mathematical science by not observing. To observation the sun moves round the earth, light things do rise and do not fall equally with lead. Modern science has led to power over Nature and to technology, but real people have been reduced to mere observers of measurements. Goethe was concerned with his vivid observations and thereafter with the ideas that arose in relation to these observations, these perceptions. Throughout Goethe's life the materialistic and mechanistic interpretation of Nature was growing in strength until it became well-nigh totally exclusive and all-powerful. Goethe and others like him considered that science had taken a false path, and he spent an immense amount of time and effort throughout his life examining and studying the multitude of detailed natural phenomena then known, on which to form the basis for his own understanding.

We need to remind ourselves sometimes of the extent to which a mechanistic view of the world has come to dominate so many of our attitudes today, and how significant areas in the work of eminent scientists and thinkers have been side-lined or indeed largely ignored. It is often forgotten that Sir Isaac Newton spent much more time and effort studying alchemy and astrology than he had spent on his recognized contributions to mechanical physics. It is also forgotten that William Harvey, discoverer of the blood circulatory system and one of the fathers of modern science, remained a life-long Aristotelian and maintained that the blood moved the heart and not vice versa. Leibniz invented the calculus, synchronously with Newton, without which modern technology would have been impossible. He was also, philosophically, one of the great line of monadologists who viewed creation as composed of quantities of individual particles, or monads. His monads, however, were not material particles but spiritual beings of varying levels of consciousness.

It is usually overlooked that the brain is an object in our consciousness which we study as any other object, rather than our consciousness a subject within the brain. Seen like this it becomes possible to consider our thoughts as only reflections in the brain, which we become conscious of just like we become conscious of our faces when we look into a mirror. But the mirror image is not the reality and Goethe sought the archetypes or Real Ideas which are the formative powers within the phenomena. He sought the 'archetypal plant', which manifested—in all the multitudinous forms of plants and their organs—that living Ideal Reality which creates the plants and which, to the extent that we can perceive it, enables us to recognize all these forms as plants.

We can approach the problem in a simplified way by thinking of a jigsaw puzzle. We can start with a whole picture and then cut it up into fragmented bits and pieces, which can be fitted together again to achieve a semblance of the picture. Alternatively, we can, like a modern scientist, start with the pieces and try to construct wholes out of them. Where, however, did those pieces originate? A 'bits-and-pieces picture' never becomes the whole that can inspire every portion with meaning, for meaning only arises in the relation of a part to the whole. The problem of the whole has haunted modern biology and even cosmology for a long time. General Smuts coined the word 'holism' and it is under this title that the problem has become popularized. It may help us if we can realize that 'wholeness' is the same as spirit or being. By its very nature wholeness cannot be grasped with the abstract concepts with which we have conquered the world of the inorganic. Modern science deals primarily with the matter that fills up the form of the living plant, animal or human being. Without this matter filling up the living plant form we should not, with our ordinary senses, be able to see the plant. Goethe trained his imaginative thinking in order to perceive this archetypal plant, his *Urpflanze*, without the help and hindrance of the matter filling up the individual plant.

It is due to the dogmatic assertion of science that only the sense-perceptible is the object of knowledge and that all else is mysticism and mere fancy, that knowledge of supersensible reality is denied to the sphere of science and relegated to the subjective realms of art and religious faith. It may however be true, as affirmed by Steiner and by many other profound thinkers of our times, that mankind is undergoing the birth pangs of a new consciousness, an imaginative consciousness, a new way of seeing that can slowly be trained to be as accurate as our old consciousness has been in its own field. The chaos of our times may well be the evidence of this new birth trauma—so let us avoid, if we can, a still birth.

The new synthetic or projective geometry of the nineteenth century (which was, incidentally, developed out of sixteenth-century studies of perspective) is already a good example of a strict training in imaginative thinking in a wide-awake consciousness—not, it must be emphasized, a dreaming consciousness. To it belongs an essential in imaginative thinking: the introduction of the principle of polarity. Contraction and expansion is one example of this, demonstrated by the polarity of point (the infinitely contracted) with the plane (the infinitely expanded). When the expanding sphere becomes, at infinity, the plane at infinity, its curvature vanishes and it becomes flat. Greece in the sixth century BC saw the passing away of the old pictorial, mythological thinking, and it must be remembered that the discovery much later of infinity in mathematics certainly heralded a dawning new consciousness.

This new geometry has also made accessible to thinking consciousness the phenomena of metamorphosis. If we shine a torch vertically downwards on the floor, the light appears as a circle. As we lift the beam it becomes an ellipse and then a parabola and hyperbola. Those forms, rigidly differentiated from each other in Euclidean geometry and the coordinate geometry of Descartes, become the metamorphoses of the archetypal so-called conic section—so-called, because if we take a cone and cut it across at different angles we get the same forms. The rigidly defined and separated forms move into each other. George Adams and Olive Whicher, in their book *The Plant Between Sun and Earth*, were able to show how the metamorphosing plant, as it grows, manifests changing forms beautifully portrayable and describable in the forms of projective geometry. The visibly portrayable metamorphoses are also mathematically thinkable, when that thinking has itself gone through a development. The coordinate geometry of René Descartes was certainly able to identify an equation with a geometric form, what we might call 'connecting a thinkable with a visible'. However, it remained tied to the rigidly defined forms of Euclid's geometry. In coordinate geometry the *thinkable* $x^2 + y^2 = r^2$ is *visible* as a circle, but with projective geometry it is possible to attain living, mobile ideas correlate with the metamorphosing forms of life, for example leaf, petal, etc. The real plant is to be found in these forms and formative forces. We can only perceive the forms with our ordinary senses because they are filled up with matter, but this matter is really only the corpse already within the living. We are faced with a radical change in our way of thinking if we are not to become imprisoned altogether in this corpse.

5. Upside-down Thinking

From time to time we really have to turn ourselves and our thinking upside down and inside out. W.H. Gaskell at the beginning of the twentieth century showed how the vertebrates are, in a sense, a turning inside out of the invertebrates. Let us consider from one point of view a possible change of paradigms in these issues.

We are accustomed to thinking of the cell as the origin of the mature organism, which is composed of a multitude of cells. But we can take a much longer view. It is easy to see that much of our mineral kingdom, mountains and so on, are the residue of once living creatures. Perhaps the whole mineral kingdom is such. Perhaps the macrocosmos as a living spiritual organism, gradually and by successive stages, brought about the precipitation of dead matter. Our skeleton could then be seen as the product of our living organism and not vice versa. We can imagine the origin of a living being, altogether human, as preceding conception. Schopenhauer thought that the unborn, unconceived child brought the parents together. Could it be that this yet preconceived child incarnates first in the warmth of the love between the parents, enters into their animated mutual life ('anima' means both soul and breath) and then participates in the fluid mixing involved in conception? This is understandable when one uses the ancient idea of the 'ether', not in the sense of nineteenth-century physicists who described it as a very fine but definitely material substance filling all space, but rather in the sense that Steiner used it, as a spiritual force that works from the periphery of space. In the planar, two-dimensional, non-Euclidian space of projective geometry, the etheric form is able to participate in the fluid realm because this realm is essentially two- not three-dimensional, as one can see when a drop of ink or milk enters water and spreads as two-dimensional veils. Having participated in conception, only then does this form begin to be filled with developing cells.

Attention has been given recently to the myriad of mites and other insects living parasitically in all the glands and follicles of our skin. We have long been familiar with worms and bacteria living parasitically in our intestines and it is quite possible to imagine all the cells in our bodies as invading parasites; our whole organism, in fact, could be seen as an ecosystem. Steiner also portrayed the human form in early evolution even before it was filled out with cells, a form probably only perceivable to Goethean or imaginative cognition. This helps one to understand how the cells themselves could then be seen as invading parasites!

Samuel Hahnemann (1755–1843) was an almost exact contemporary of Goethe (1749–1832) and pioneered a revolutionary new form of medicine, homoeopathy, which has continued as a minority movement until today. It has been misunderstood and derided by officialdom in much the same way as has Goethe's science. Goethe was interested in this new development in medicine and it is recorded that he himself consulted a homoeopathic physician.

What is generally known about this system is its use of greatly diluted remedies. They are so diluted that in the higher dilutions, commonly used, no molecule of the original substance could be present. Therefore, in the views of those trained in modern materialistic science and medicine, it is obviously nonsense. However if one approaches the problem with the help of projective geometry and not with one-sidedly Euclidean geometry, then with the rhythmically repeated dilution and succussion (a shaking called potentizing) it becomes understandable that the substance could be raised from its almost material state backwards through its evolutionary development to its etheric (or planar geometric) origin. The Goethean Idea of the remedial substance is released. This understanding was most beautifully set forth by Adams.

The use of potentized substances as remedies is only one aspect of Hahnemann's contribution. He also contrasted the phenomena of acute and chronic diseases or, speaking broadly, of inflammatory and sclerotic processes. Acute, inflammatory diseases, typical of childhood, move towards self-healing. In Hahnemann's day they occurred in epidemics but now, in the so-called developed world, childhood illnesses have been largely eliminated by immunization programmes. In the so-called Third World, however, they still wreak havoc amongst the undernourished children who are also weakened by malaria, tuberculosis and parasitic infestations. Inflammations are characterized by heat, pain, swelling and redness, which are still taught under the old names Calor, Dolor, Tumor and Rubor. These four features or symptoms of inflammation recall the four elements and humours of Greek times: Calor is the Fire; Dolor, the pain, actually experienced in the soul or anima, is the element of Air; Tumor, the swelling, is the watery manifestation; and in the redness, Rubor, the expression comes into the material earthy element. The processes of inflammation arise in response to foreign invasion of the organism by bacteria or other foreign bodies. The process brings it about that the invading entity is digested and the residue eliminated as pus or other excrement or as the rashes of childhood illnesses. The integrity or wholeness of the organism is restored and in successful cases is even strengthened and achieves a new, higher, level of development.

We can approach this type of disease process in many ways. For our purpose now, we can see it as a metamorphosis of the normal processes of digestion. We take in foreign substance as food and digest it. It has to be broken down completely before it can be resurrected in the bloodstream and used to build up the organism. Digestion is actually a *normal* inflammation process and the faeces can be seen metamorphically in the same light as the pus of an abscess. When inflammatory or digestive processes occur *outside* the intestine then we regard it as an illness.

Polar to these inflammatory or acute diseases are the hardening or sclerotic diseases of ageing. As the body grows older it grows harder, less elastic, and eventually at death it is cast off to disintegrate. To these ageing diseases, which occur mostly in the second half of life, belong the diseases of hardened arteries, osteo-arthritis, cataracts in the eyes and degenerative diseases of the nervous system. It is in the nervous system that we can find the archetype of these diseases. It is characteristic of the brain and spinal cord that nerve cells are dying off from birth onwards and any capacity for renewal of nerve cells is absent or extremely limited. Whereas the cells lining our intestines multiply many times faster than the cells of the most malignant tumour, those of the brain can, after birth, only die off.

Steiner repeatedly drew attention to two polar forms of evil, which he referred to under the names of Lucifer and Ahriman. Lucifer is connected with the serpent in the Garden of Eden and Mephistopheles in Goethe's *Faust* is mostly a portrayal of Ahriman. In the Old Testament Book of Job these two forces, two spiritual beings, appear as Leviathan and Behemoth. Evil and sin resulting from the luciferic influence carry an inherent tendency to repentance and recovery. The suffering resultant from it propels towards metanoia, 'change of mind', the Greek for repentance. The ahrimanic evil carries no such impulse. We must meet it with a higher self-awakening and self-engendered rising into freedom of thought and action. Through this, meaning can be conferred on the otherwise meaningless evil.

The human being has to establish a place midway between the two evils, and a correspondence of these two can be made with the first polarity in illness which Hahnemann emphasized: the acute, inflammatory diseases (luciferic in nature), which have similarities to the digestion process and which tend to self-healing, and the chronic, sclerotic diseases (ahrimanic in nature), which are a metamorphosis of the brain and nervous processes which lead to chronic deterioration with no self-healing.

Hahnemann also emphasized a second polarity. He pointed out that most patients consulting a physician have symptoms, some of them mental or emotional and some of them bodily and local. He characterized the most difficult: for example, all the disorder manifests in local disturbance whilst the patient remains mentally sound; or all the disorder appears in a disturbance of the thoughts, emotions or the will to action, whilst a local organic basis remains difficult to find. Characteristic of the diseases appearing in a local anatomical manifestation are all the tumour-forming illnesses culminating in cancers of various types, whereas the 'mental' diseases culminate in schizophrenia and the psychoses. It is only with difficulty that one can discover psychological abnormality in cancer patients or find local lesions at the basis of the psychoses.

The Bahnsons, the American psychiatrist couple who, in 1963, made a study of psychosomatic aspects of neoplastic disease (cancer), posited a polarity of disease from cancer to deteriorated psychosis, with a spectrum or seesaw in between. From the centre pivot, on one side hysteria progressed to anxiety hysteria, anxiety states, obsessional and phobic states, and compulsive neuroses to paranoid psychoses and finally to deteriorated psychoses (or schizophrenia). On the other side hysteria progressed to conversion hysteria to hypochondriasis, psychosomatic conditions to organic diseases of the gastro-intestinal, respiratory and circulatory systems and finally to cancer. The polarity of cancer and schizophrenia appears with the spectrum of diseases in between. (The individual patient, of course, does not progress through these stages, which represent only an attempt at a systematic classification.) This seems to me to be a distinct second polarity after that of the acute inflammatory diseases polar to the chronic sclerotic diseases.

A further polarity can help to bring order and understanding into the bewildering labyrinth of diseases which face us, and which today tend to be treated each as a separate entity. At the end of the nineteenth century neurasthenia and hysteria were commonly described and even contrasted. Neurasthenia was the name given to conditions characterized by fatigue, headache, backache and oversensitivity to sensory stimuli. Various other names have been given to similar symptoms during the last two centuries which would now cover many cases of chronic fatigue syndrome. Hysteria, also, had been highlighted and over-dramatized by Charcot at the Saltpetrière hospital, but gradually the use of these names faded from popularity. Steiner was able to deepen the understanding of the processes signified by these names. He pointed to a current of so-called 'astral forces' that passed from the head down the spinal cord. These must be understood as a system of forces belonging to the animal level, or we could say the soul or consciousness level of the human organism, which have a great deal of influence in the realm of the emotions. Their organic manifestation can be traced from evolutionary and embryological phenomena onwards.

Let me include a few words on this. Animal development, as distinct from vegetable development, proceeds by processes of invagination (in-turning). Instead of the typical planar, exteriorizing growth of the plant, we find an interiorizing gesture in the animal. By this means an inside and outside come into existence, by infolding or pushing in. Instead of a continued growth outwards in space as in the plant, growth is held back and turned inwards. In this way animal forms appear through a kind of sculpturing or modelling process, and thereby these 'astral' forces or 'forces of soul' are revealed as being also a source of form. Animal forms can now be seen in the human being, as the physiognomy of different characters within the soul. For instance, the fox is revealed as the physiognomy of cunning, the lion of courage.

In 1785, the German physicist Chladni observed that if one took a metal plate, covered it with fine sand or powder and, by stroking it with a violin bow brought it into vibrating, singing music, then the sand danced into forms. Most complex forms and movements have been made visible in this way and help us to grasp that music creates form. Music, widely acknowledged as the language of the soul, gives rise not only to dance but also to forms, even the forms of animal organs. The music of the spheres is the higher reality of what Steiner called astral or soul forces. These astral forces have a strong connection with the nervous system and when we look at the spinal cord descending through the vertebrae and see the nerves radiating out, particularly around the chest, it is not difficult to picture this as a musical instrument, such as the lyre beloved by Apollo.

Let us follow the movement of these sculpturing, but destructive catabolic forces through the spinal cord. In normal conditions they pass to the kidneys and are there diverted to radiate, as what Steiner called the 'kidney radiation', into the organism. Here they function as animating forces arousing the nutritional stream in the blood from merely living into a feeling and mobile existence. It may happen that these forces are cramped in the brain and spinal cord and only in diminished quantity reach to the realm of the kidney. Then arises the neurasthenic state, headache, backache, over-sensitivity and weakened nutrition and weakened ensouling of the body. It is suggested that this 'kidney radiation' is to some extent caught by the suprarenal glands, which sit like hats on the kidneys, and then works in the adrenal hormones. (It is interesting also that early on in embryonic development the kidneys originate at the head pole of the body and from there descend to the abdomen, moving from pronephros, i.e., the kidney in the region of the ear, to mesonephros, i.e., the kidney descended to the urogenital organs, to metanephros and the final placing of the kidneys in the abdomen of the developed foetus.)

On the other hand, these descending astral forces may be diverted in the kidneys, radiate into the organism but then 'leak through' some organ and escape. Instead of animating, ensouling the organism they leak away and become unconscious or semi-conscious organs of perception, reaching into the unconscious realms of other people. In this way can arise all the disturbing influences that are associated with hysteria. In neurasthenia these forces are cramped, imprisoned in the brain and spinal cord, whereas in hysteria they escape into the environment. Speaking generally, the neurasthenic tends to look prematurely old, the hysteric remains youthful looking.

We can now look at the relationship between these three polarities of disease tendencies and the three dimensions of our bodies: upwards and downwards, backwards and forwards, left and right. For example, we walk forwards into the future and leave the past behind us, and the acute diseases typical of childhood mark steps into the future whilst the sclerotic diseases of ageing show the dominance of the past behind us.

Concerning the up and down polarity, Steiner gave a most fruitful suggestion that in cancerous diseases a sense organ (more especially the ear) is trying to establish itself in a metabolic organ. A metabolic organ, for instance the stomach, is trying to become an ear or sense organ. (I remember two patients with cancers of the stomach who told me that they tasted their food in the stomach.) Steiner points to another expression of the up and down polarity in psychoses where consciousness is overwhelmed by the premature eruption of some content of the unconscious into consciousness. From the realm of the metabolic organs below, the unprepared consciousness (in the head pole) is invaded by disturbing manifestations which could be, at a later time and after preparation, *healthy* phenomena. The patient does not know what to make of a soul content that really belongs to some future time. It can be understood as something from the past, buried in the unconscious, awaiting resurrection in some future but bursting through prematurely into the present.

The neurasthenic and hysteric polarity has a left and right nature characterized in the blood circulation. The red arterial blood goes out from the heart on the left side whereas the blue venous blood returns on the right. This relates to how the hysteric tendency to escape, to flow out, is more noticeable on the left. Hysterical paralyses and anaesthesias are more marked on the left side, the neurasthenic cramping is more right-sided. We know that the left side of the body is related to the right side of the human brain and the right side of the body to the left brain. Further we know that the left brain is related to verbal and abstract thinking, the right brain to poetry, music and the feelings. The parallels are clear. I think we can also glimpse a meaning in the fact that whereas in mammals the aorta rising up from the heart arches over to the left, in birds it arches over to the right. Poppelbaum, in his book *Man and Animal,* showed how in birds the whole body is metamorphosed into a head. He saw birds as 'heads' flying around, and we have only to watch to see how more awake they are than dreaming animals such as carnivores and ruminants. If mammals can be seen as incarnated emotions then may not birds be seen as incarnated thoughts, the soaring philosophic thoughts of the eagle and the streetwise thoughts of the cockney sparrows? Left and right in mammals are *reversed* in the human head and in birds. Through these experiences of polarity we can gradually work our way towards a grasp of diseases as metamorphoses of healthy processes. We can more easily see the repeated falling into disease and the ever-renewed healing as a necessary continuous process. Health as a state is actually an illusion, but healing can bring about a real progress in the evolution of the human being towards spiritual perfection.

We must go beyond Hahnemann's vision that the physician's task was to restore the patient to the state of health he was in before he fell ill. That is a static view of a human being, who changes and develops throughout life and should grow and keep growing not just physically but in soul and spirit. In walking we fall to the left and then to the right but keep our balance or restore it continuously as we walk towards our goal. What is our goal? Merely to prolong a seemingly meaningless existence is an unworthy goal of any truly modern medicine. Nietzsche put forward the goal of Superman but, unfortunately, this has been interpreted materialistically as some new biological development. Nor can the goal of humanity only be to become 'a good man' as envisaged by ordinary morality, but rather the fulfilment, the perfecting of all the potentialities lying latent or repressed in our nature. In the progress towards our goal, disease and its healing should be major contributors.

6. Dogs, Snakes and Mirrors

Hahnemann's main contributions were, firstly, to see that 'disease' comes to expression in the totality of symptoms. We cannot reach the reality of a disease by our current chemical and physical studies which only grasp the corpse of the living, for the living reality, he maintained, is expressed in the symptoms. Here disease is obviously understood as an 'Idea' in the Goethean sense and Imagination is called for to grasp the Idea manifesting in the symptoms. Secondly, Hahnemann then observed that similar symptoms could arise in response to poisonings by substances whether accidentally or experimentally given, so-called 'provings'. He then found that a substance bringing about a complex of symptoms in a normally healthy person would act remedially when given to a patient with similar symptoms. (Paracelsus suggested that diseases should be classified by their remedies. For example, all the different diseases for which sulphur could be the remedy should be named together as Sulphur disease.) Hahnemann conjectured that the new disease given by the remedy would block the naturally occurring disease. Such a view is the reverse of that of Hippocrates, for whom the symptoms were the expression of Nature's healing efforts. Both views could lead to treatment by 'likes' but for opposite reasons. It seems to me that we must look at both from the context of the changed consciousness and changed constitution of the human being in the intervening two thousand years.

In Greece, Hippocrates was working at the twilight of the fading old oriental spiritual culture, in which the spiritual in Nature, the Goddess, was still to some extent perceived. Hahnemann's work came fairly early in the developing, materialistically orientated Western culture. Nature was becoming understood as mechanical and, for the new consciousness, 'purpose' in Nature was taboo. The idea of blocking a disease by giving a similar one certainly underlies a very great deal of modern chemical drugs, but the disease is grasped on a molecular level and the remedy is engineered as a similar molecule to the one on the diseased pathway. In such a way the individual patient vanishes from view, for the sophisticated statistical methods designed to assess treatment deliberately eliminate the individual. Hahnemann like Goethe stuck with the perceptible, rejecting all the dawning chemistry and physics, electricity and magnetism which do not belong to the visible and perceptible. For Goethe the Idea of the archetypal plant *was* imaginatively perceptible, and his concept of metamorphosis in plants can easily be extended to the world of insects. Picture for a moment the butterfly. From egg to caterpillar to chrysalis to the butterfly, the insect ascends as does the plant from seed to stem with leaves, to calyx from which bursts forth the butterfly blossom. In the plant we see the metamorphosis simultaneously and sequentially, whereas in the insect it is only sequential. Metamorphosis in the insect may be arrested at an early stage, e.g. at the leaf stage as in the leaf insects.

Steiner pointed to another metamorphosis, this time within the human being. He demonstrated how some of the forces of growth active in the organism during the first seven years of life then become metamorphosed into the forces with which we think. We think with the same forces with which we were earlier forming our growing body. As we grow older, further levels of organizing activities are liberated into the conscious soul functions, most obviously the emotional at puberty.

Hahnemann's fundamental idea about treatment with 'likes' can now be approached with these metamorphic insights. The medicinal plant, for instance, can be grasped with such Goethean ideas as it undergoes a higher metamorphosis when taken into the human organism. We need to bring our imaginative idea of, say, monkshood (*Aconitum napellus*) into so flexible a state that we can see it again in full expression in the 'drug picture', the poisoning symptoms of Aconite. This is not fundamentally more difficult than perceiving the future red admiral in its caterpillar stage. In both cases we need the sensory perceptions as well as the imaginative Idea.

How can we now understand the action of the remedy in the healing process? Firstly, we have suggested that we must see the image of the remedy in the 'potentized' form. How can a mere image act therapeutically? We all know that a look in the mirror in the morning can often serve to change one's consciousness and even, occasionally, one's lifestyle! Cannot the unreality, the imagination of a play for example, produce profound results? Shakespeare's Hamlet certainly found that this was so:

O, what a rogue and peasant slave am I!
Is it not monstrous that this player here,
But in a fiction, in a dream of passion,
Could force his soul so to his own conceit
That from her working all his visage wann'd;
Tears in his eyes, distraction in's aspect,
A broken voice, and his whole function suiting

With forms to his conceit? And all for nothing!
For Hecuba!

Hamlet (Act 2, Scene ii)

When we realize that the human being is a compendium of all nature, as Jaworski showed, then we can glimpse that such a plant remedy would be able to activate those of its corresponding processes to be found in the human organism, and that even its image alone may serve to vary the level of consciousness of such interiorized functions or organs within the human organism. In this way, for instance, some buried content, lost beyond the threshold of consciousness, may be made more accessible. In the case of Aconite it is often fear or fright that, when repressed, gives rise to the whole range of the symptoms. The full healing process, however, calls for the yet further integration of the repressed content by conscious effort, in addition to the freeing of this lost event or trauma from its burial ground.

Hahnemann was aware and appreciative of the growing interest in mesmerism and hypnotism in his time—a sphere of interest that ultimately gave rise to the modern psychology of the unconscious in its manifold expressions. Amongst the early psychoanalysts of the 1920s it was in particular Georg Groddeck who showed that the methods and insights of this new approach were most effective in the treatment of so-called organic diseases. I am now suggesting that the potentized immaterial homoeopathic remedy, as mirror image of the original plant or other source of the remedy, changes the consciousness and awakens from sleep some corresponding process or element in the disease phenomena. I remember that Fritz Künkel, another leading psychiatrist of those days, suggested that the healing effect in those early talking cures came about when a 'mirror' was held up to the patient, so that he could see himself as others see him. He emphasized that this must not be done too soon, else the effect could be shattering.

I think that we can get some help in entering into these unusual ways of looking at illness and its healing by recalling the ancient symbols of the healing process. In ancient Greece, healing was looked upon as the epiphany, the manifestation, of the god Asclepius. Whether the healing came about through the vision of the god as the patient lay in 'temple sleep', or through a physician whose blood bore the inheritance from Asclepius (the divine ancestor of the tribe of physicians), it was in the healing process that the god was seen to incarnate. We mentioned earlier that Asclepius was always accompanied by attendant animals, snakes and dogs, whose lick therapy was an acknowledged treatment. In the museum at the Roman baths in Bath, England, there is an altar to Aesculapius (the Roman name for Asclepius) and on one side is a snake, on another a dog. In Venice one comes upon the interesting story of San Rocco, a patron saint of the plague, who himself became infected while caring for victims of bubonic plague, but was then cured when his dog licked the ulcers. Thereafter San Rocco always took his dog with him and wherever we find pictures of the saint he is always portrayed with his dog. Another symbolic aspect of the dog is as guard dog, protector of thresholds. There is even an icon of St Christopher who carried the Christ child across a river, where the head of the saint is actually a dog's head. In Goethe's *Faust* the manifestations of Mephistopheles are invariably heralded by his poodle.

Now the bite of a mad dog can cause rabies, that terrible disease which brings on spasms of the throat. What is the throat? The region of the throat and neck is where we swallow from the conscious realm of taste and smell into the unconscious realm of forgetfulness. It is the gateway through which we vomit or regurgitate from forgetfulness back into consciousness. Further, it is where the nasal passages cross over from back to front in order to continue down the larynx and trachea into the lungs, whilst the mouth crosses over to the back to pass down the gullet into the stomach. It is also the region where left and right interchange in the spinal cord. Common speech talks about getting the neck of someone or some problem, and executioners hang, or throttle, or cut off the head with axe or guillotine. How are snakes and dogs related to all this? We have noted how dogs are very much connected with thresholds, and the throat is obviously such a threshold between an upper world and the underworld of the belly. For the Greeks, it was the three-headed dog Cerberus that one would encounter by the River Styx, at the frontier of the underworld.

We have a wonderful example of the snake nature from South Africa, where there is a small egg-eating snake that has spikes from its vertebrae in the region behind the head penetrating into the oesophagus. When it eats an egg whose size is greater than itself, it crushes the egg against these spikes and sends the egg down into the stomach and the shell is regurgitated upwards. Remembering and forgetting, we can swallow some insults down but others stick in our gullet. Some things need to be remembered, others forgotten. This snake gives us a picture of how to do this, and encourages us to ponder as to whether the realm of the forgotten, from which memories must be awoken, is actually the underworld of the organs of the *body* rather than the brain in the head.

This latter is where we become conscious again when memory awakens.

These considerations, however far they may seem from our medical problems of today, can help us to win imaginations for the medicine of the future. Snakes are traditionally linked with Lucifer and the dog with Mephistopheles, or Ahriman as Steiner called him. Between these forces of evil waiting at the threshold of the human soul we must continuously re-establish our balance.

7. Miasms and Moral Challenge

For our present purposes we can still find in the legacy of
Samuel Hahnemann a further riddle and germinal idea for
the future. His earlier work dealt mostly with acute, feverish
illnesses, diseases such as scarlet fever, smallpox, measles.
These were all epidemic and, with dysenteries and diar-
rhoeas and pneumonias, killed numberless young people
and children. They are mostly the kind of illnesses that run a
typical course and end in death or recovery. Such illness is
also in some sense a healing or leads inherently to the
awakening of healing forces. In his later years Hahnemann
became more involved in chronic diseases, the diseases more
characteristic of ageing and old age. These diseases, which in
our so-called developed world have become more important,
are the ones that show little tendency to self-healing. They
run a long, progressive course and today manifest as diseases
of the heart and blood vessels, diseases of the nervous system
and dementias, and as the varied realm of tumour form-
ations, cancers and the like, which affect mostly the metabolic
and reproductive organs. Hahnemann must have found
himself up against more difficult problems, as has everyone
else, in trying to heal these diseases. His insistence that the
disease comes to expression in the totality of symptoms, *is* that
totality itself, becomes almost unworkable because the
symptoms of 20 or more years ago, at the beginning of the
disease, are forgotten or distorted in memory. Hahnemann
came up with ideas about these chronic diseases which have
sown seeds of controversy amongst his followers ever since.

He characterized three archetypal diseases, or 'miasms' of

the dynamic unity of the organism, in other words, the 'being' of the sick person. To these he gave names which have probably led to misunderstandings ever since. He called them Syphilis, Psora and Sycosis. Now I think that by Syphilis he meant not simply the disease we today define as syphilis, but rather the whole constitutional, underlying state that enables the disease we call syphilis to take hold and manifest. The symptoms are far wider in mental and constitutional directions. Again, by Psora he meant a much broader picture than the itch of scabies which was then so common. Sycosis, manifesting in mucous discharges and warty growths, was not *just* gonorrhoea. This latter could develop in a constitution already predisposed by Sycosis. These three Hahnemannian conceptions cannot be understood as material entities but are best grasped as Goethean Ideas, real forces graspable by imaginative thinking, artistic picture forming. I touch on these somewhat technical aspects of the homoeopathic tradition because I believe this will help us to attain a better insight into our present medical problems.

From the fifteenth century we can trace the development of our modern intellectual and scientific consciousness. One of the hallmarks of this way of thinking, the scientific and experimental method, is that it separates its pursuit of truth from all emotional, and from all moral and religious mixture or contamination. In previous ages Truth, Beauty and Goodness or Science, Art and Religion were aspects of one whole reality which therefore could obviously not be solely material or sensory. The extreme separation of the sensory material world from the supersensible worlds of soul and spirit lay in the future. Francis Bacon, Lord Verulam (1561– 1626), one of the early protagonists of this new conscious- ness, maintained that one could think anything without its interfering with one's religious faith. Thinking was becoming autonomous. Interestingly enough, at the turn of the sixteenth century, after Columbus's return from the Caribbean, a pandemic of the disease syphilis spread over Europe almost immediately. From our present point of view it is not important whether Columbus imported the disease from the West or not. The disease may or may not have occurred occasionally before. What does seem certain is that it now became pandemic, and I am suggesting that this is related to the new intellectual thinking, freed from feeling and moral or religious values. As a disease, syphilis can attack any of the tissues and organs of the body but its most central attack does seem to be on the brain and nervous system, the very instruments of thinking. As this new thinking took hold it became attacked by a disease that appeared synchronously, and I suggest that this whole complex of purely intellectual thinking, based exclusively on sense data, comes nearer to the Ideal perceived imaginatively by Hahnemann under the name Syphilis. The disease was the price paid for the new consciousness which has led to our technologically dominated world.

When this new consciousness began to appear and, with Copernicus, Galileo and Newton, assumed direction of scientific research there was an upsurge of optimism. The Royal Society was formed and men looked forward to the conquest of Nature, poverty and ignorance. However it was not to be. The Thirty Years War was unleashed and Central Europe was devastated for a hundred years. Disillusionment was widespread and people began to look to idealism in social reform and to poetic romanticism as the way forward. In place of what we might call 'thinking thinking', which was often aphoristic, and inclined to philosophic poetry, there developed a more 'dreaming thinking' and romantic poetry. Of course these tendencies co-existed and interpenetrated, but they are there to see. Together with the earliest beginnings of the Industrial Revolution there developed the romanticism of Coleridge, Wordsworth, Keats and many others. Blake sought the New Jerusalem amidst the dark satanic mills and was an explicit opponent of Newton's mechanistic physics. Gradually art, which had been wedded to religion and ancient cosmology, became emancipated. Secular themes became as much subject for artistic depiction as religious ones and with these changes there came about the pandemic of tuberculosis. Now tuberculosis had been with us throughout recorded history. Mummies from Egypt have been shown to have had tuberculous lesions and the Greeks gave excellent accounts of its symptoms. In the eighteenth and nineteenth centuries in Europe it assumed epidemic proportions and scarcely a family but had a member dying of consumption, the wasting disease. Many sanitoria were opened to care for the sufferers and Thomas Mann in *The Magic Mountain* gave a wonderful depiction of the psycho-social life within them. Now this disease also can affect any organ, but its most typical, characteristic expression is in the lungs. Here we have the centre of the rhythmic processes within the organism that mediate between and balance those polar forces centred in the head and the abdomen, i.e., in the nerve-sense and metabolic-limb processes, which are centred in head and belly but all-pervasive throughout. Within the homoeopathic school tuberculosis has often been recognized as an expression of Hahnemann's Psoric miasm, even as its *most* typical form. Psora can then be understood as a disturbance in the actual self-healing processes themselves. That some homoeopathic physicians sought to identify this Psora with 'original sin' is perhaps understandable.

The third of Hahnemann's miasms he called Sycosis. Hahnemann reached these formative ideas out of a life-long study of the symptoms of disease in all their multi-tudinous variety and detail just as Goethe reached his *Urpflanze* out of an enormous study of the details of plant growth. This idea Sycosis found its expression typically in disorders of the mucous membranes, the inner linings of the organs, and in a range of warty and tumour form-ations. Mucous discharges were an expression, and in an age when syphilis and gonorrhoea were very widespread venereal diseases this Sycosis was frequently identified with gonorrhoea. Indicative symptoms were observed by homoe-opathic physicians treating these disorders. The Syphilitic type of patient was observed to prefer the mountains whilst the Sycotic type was better at the seaside. Further, the symptoms of the Syphilitic type were often worse at night whilst the Sycotic preferred the night to the day. One might also bear in mind the similarities that suggest them-selves when we consider fear and shame as a polarity. Fear is a feeling often associated with darkness, whereas shame burns more strongly when exposed to the light of day. Fear drains the blood from the face and makes one feel frozen to the spot; shame brings the blood to the face and makes one long to vanish from the spot, to flow out on the heat of the blood and disappear into the void. Fear is an intense nerve experience; shame is an experience of being over-whelmed with the forces of the blood.

Such symptoms can open more doors to a fuller under-standing of disease than our prevailing materialistic con-cepts. Here we are, yet again, dealing with polarity.

Hahnemann's Syphilis and Sycosis are the polar opposites and his Psora is the disease of the very balancing, healing mercurial function itself. Syphilis is related more to the ectodermally derived tissues, Sycosis to those derived predominantly from the endoderm and Psora to those originated from the mesoderm.

In the middle of the nineteenth century another change took place in both the prevailing social and psychological realms. The social idealism of the earlier part of the century had failed to control the industrial revolution with its degradation of the masses to the status of wage slaves. Marxism appeared and demanded planning and organization for the Revolution. All traditional moral values were queried: Nietzsche exposed them as the Will to Power of ruling classes; Dostoevsky's characters claimed that 'to the superior man all things are permitted'. Action became divorced from all moral and aesthetic values. So now we had the thinking, the feeling and the will progressively and successively emancipated, and mutually isolated from each other. What is now the medical price of this freedom? Tuberculosis began to wane and its place was taken by cancer in its varied forms. Cancer mainly attacks the organs of the metabolic-limb and reproductive systems. The will is related to the metabolic-limb system as feeling is to the rhythmic system and thinking to the nerve-sense system. The American psychiatrist G. Booth, who worked in the 1950s, was able to show that the psychological characteristics of tuberculosis patients, as revealed in the Rorschag 'ink blot' tests, corresponded to the ruling social values that prevailed in the early nineteenth century. The same tests given to cancer patients revealed social values more typical of the twentieth century. The psychological character of tuberculosis was the social

norm of the nineteenth century, that of cancer the norm of
the century following.

We can see how the disintegration of ancient mutuality of
thinking, feeling and will is expressed in the wider cultural
life. Scientific thinking became inartistic, non-religious,
amoral. Art, which was in earlier times wedded to religious
themes and images, turned first to the portrayal of secular
scenes and then became freed from any tendency even to
realism. Art has striven to establish its own realm, art for art's
sake, separated from both the portrayal of an outer, natural
reality and from the imaging of the spiritual realities of the
supersensory realms. Religion has become conventional
morality divorced from both art and cosmology.

If in earlier times evolution was always guided and
balanced by the wisdom of a divine world, which could in
scientific terminology be called the world of the unconscious, then it is so no longer. Today, this separation of
science, art and religion or of thinking, feeling and will can
only be balanced and healed by the conscious activity of the
individuality itself, or what Steiner called the ego. In the
inner experiences of individuals who have followed esoteric
paths of development, it has been known that a crisis had to
be encountered, a crossing of the threshold between this
earthly world of sense experience and the spiritual world. It
has always been known, by those able to judge, that such a
critical point was fraught with great danger if someone came
unprepared to this inner crisis. For at such a moment the ego
is called upon to rise to responsibilities of self-guidance
which hitherto it has left to God and his religious repre-
sentatives, or else to the compulsions of secular authorities.
Moral challenges face us today for which our habitual store
of concepts developed from the natural world is totally

inadequate. If we are weak in the face of such new challenges, it is hardly surprising that we are met with new diseases.

In latter years we have been experiencing an increase in so-called allergic diseases, notably asthma, hay fever and eczema, and a great deal of attention has also been focused on the so-called auto-immune diseases and HIV and AIDS, where the immune system is attacked and destroyed, and death results.

In the allergic diseases we get the picture of some outer substance that has penetrated too deeply into the organism, so that something which should have remained very much on the surface in the sphere of sensation has penetrated inside and provoked the allergic reaction. The auto-immune diseases give us a somewhat different picture of an organ or tissue that has fallen out of the wholeness of the organism, that has almost become outer world or non-self. Then the 'wholeness' reacts with greater or lesser intensity and seeks, mainly through inflammatory processes, to cook and reintegrate or eliminate what has become the foreign element. What we know as the immune system is a function of the blood system (the system described by Steiner as the 'physical seat' of the spiritual ego), and is the organic expression of self or 'wholeness' in relation to the outer or non-self. We can tentatively suggest that it is an inability of the individuality forces to discriminate between self and non-self that allows the outer to become inner or the inner to become outer. In fact such discrimination is one of the major tasks of these forces of individuality, which we also call the ego or self. Today all these processes are subjected to extreme reductionist study and the molecular level of mechanism tends to be regarded as the sole reality in the processes. We are, however, led to see in these phenomena indications that the self as an immaterial organizing force has become weakened and cannot maintain the wholeness of the organism, causing self and non-self to come into confusion. This general weakness of the capacities of ego or self arises, I am suggesting, at the historic moment when thinking, feeling and will have become separated from and independent of each other.

8. The Human Being—An Indefinite Article

In previous times the individuality was sustained to a great extent by group, race, nation, class, religion, family and so on, in varying degrees. Its attitudes to life and reality were carried by the conventions accepted in the group concerned. Individuals seldom rose to issues of independent moral and intellectual decision. During the trials of the twentieth century individuals have been experiencing an increasing isolation and loneliness, as they face the new moral dilemmas brought forth by the rapid advance of scientific technology. The achievements of reproductive technology have awoken us to burdens of moral responsibilities beyond the dreams of our ancestors. Organ transplantation, made possible with the suppression of the immune processes against the 'foreign' organ, raises the deepest questions about the relation of the self to the body in which it is incorporated. What does it mean that a point of self-consciousness, a self, finds itself in a particular body immunologically distinct from every other body? What does it mean to be born?

It has become customary in our civilization and culture to assume that the individual person comes into existence at birth or conception as a new creation. As we have mentioned, this view can be traced back to Aristotle for whom each individual person was a unique new creation but also immortal; there was no pre-existence, only post-mortem existence. These assumptions have engendered grievous moral issues today in relationship to test-tube babies, embryological research involving the killing of multitudes of fertilized ova, and abortions of 'undesirable' or unwanted foetuses. When can it be said that a human individuality is present? Norman Ford, a Catholic theologian, in his book *When did I begin?*, attempted to answer this question using all the available scientific knowledge, critically examined with the tools of Thomistic scholarship. He noted that a fertilized ovum can become divided into two up to 14 days after fertilization, and then develop into identical twins. He took this observation as decisive. An individual obviously cannot be divisible into two, one person cannot become two persons. Therefore, one cannot speak about an individuality being present before 14 days after conception at the earliest. This is not to say that the individuality is present thereafter.

Can we approach this question afresh without the accepted convention or dogma that the new-born or conceived child is an altogether novel creation. We enter this world at birth and leave it at death. Where we come from and where we go to is veiled from us in our present awake consciousness. Various phenomena occurring today indicate that in our dream and sleep consciousness we do live in another world. Many people have experienced, for instance, that a problem totally insoluble one evening is miraculously solved during sleep. On another level there are the many reports of so-called near-death experiences. Such phenomena only highlight the polarity of the spiritual and physical worlds. It is exceedingly difficult for modern individuals to form any idea of the spiritual. It is difficult enough for most modern people to grasp the reality of the *soul*, let alone of the spirit. For four hundred years the natural-scientific viewpoint has insisted that only what can be weighed and measured is 'real'. The actual soul *experience* of quality in colour, taste, tone, smell, etc. are relegated to the forbidden realm of the occult as Owen Barfield has shown. Thoughts are now increasingly affirmed to be products of the brain. Feelings are taken, even by William James the American psychologist and pragmatist, as simply the perception of changed physiological processes. Free will has become a delusion; only a sort of reflex action exists. Man has become automaton.

It belongs to the commonly accepted dogmas of our natural-scientific establishment that the human being is a part of Nature, and that Nature is the Whole. Nature is understood as either determined by unchanging laws, such as the law of conservation of matter, or else a chaos out of which order is supposed to emerge. In either case there is no room for the moral world order, yet the question remains: would the human being be human without that basic morality that we sense in our conscience?

Nature has been represented as the realm of the finite. This implies limitation both in space and time, one thing is not another; things are separated from each other down to the notion of atoms or subatomic entities. Over against this realm of the finite we have to posit the realm of the Infinite. It belongs to the discoveries of synthetic, i.e., projective, geometry to have revealed that infinity is not just a large number, it is not a number at all. Number belongs to the realm of the finite, of separateness; infinity is all inclusive, without separateness. The infinitely large sphere becomes a plane. If, in imagination, we go over a sphere we come back again; in the case of a plane at infinity we come back from any direction as it were from the other side. The customary distinctions between front and back, left and right, top and bottom, vanish. Everything mutually interpenetrates everything else—separateness vanishes. If we were to say that the finite is the realm of the separated, alienated or, I should like to use Gutkind's phrase, 'hate-divided' things, then the

Infinite would be the realm of the 'love-united'. Can we get an inkling of the spiritual world as against this our natural, physical world, by taking the spiritual as the world of the Infinite and of love, and this world as the world of the finite and of alienation? The human being stands between as the realm of the indefinite, the intermediary between God and Nature. At last we can replace the dogma of Nature as Whole.

This is very different from the cultural prejudices of today which first of all regard men and women as merely specimens of the animal kingdom, while the various scientific disciplines, at the same time, seem to reduce all the kingdoms of Nature to the mineral. Molecular biology, for instance, attempts to reduce all life phenomena to molecules. Yet the human being participates in the spiritual as well as in the natural. However, it has to be said that the three natural kingdoms are certainly all rooted in the earthly, the finite, the limited. As Steiner indicated, the living plant and the animated, ensouled animal are able to become visible to us on the sensory level because these forms (themselves supersensory) are impregnated by the dead mineral stuff. All that is studied in molecular biology and in all biochemistry is only the corpse that fills up the forms. And we ourselves, we humans, are again visible to each other on the plane of our sensory perception only because we carry our corpses along with us, filling out with dead matter our immaterial spiritual forms.

It can be difficult for us, today, to begin to turn our ideas inside out as it were. We have been so indoctrinated for five centuries now with the dictat that only the weighable, measurable, touchable are real that we often quail before the challenge that the times present to our thinking. Goethe pioneered the metamorphosis of his vision into the level of consciousness that Steiner characterized as Imagination. With Imagination it becomes possible to 'see' the living, metamorphosing Idea of the plant. We cannot see this with our ordinary eyes because our eyes only see the dead matter. Imagination is a higher development of vision and it is possible for this potential faculty, latent in all of us, to be cultivated until it becomes an accurate and true faculty of knowledge. Only then will the living Idea, the archetype of the plant become visible for us. We would enter the realm of the *living* which, from another side, has been opened to us through projective geometry.

Our eye and ear are polar opposites to each other. The eye has grown outward from the brain and, as Plato could still perceive, an 'etheric limb' extends outwards to feel what we see. The ear, with its three little bones, can also be imagined as a limb but withdrawn into the depths of the cavities in the skull bones. To listen properly we have to make space, become inwardly empty, and then into this space the other can sound. Just as vision can be developed into Imagination, so can hearing be developed into what Steiner called Inspiration (he characterized these words with the greatest care). To complete the picture, a higher development of thinking leads to Intuition with which faculty one can experience another ego in the same way as one's own self-consciousness. The human being is by no means a finished article—the road to perfection is longer than we think.

I have had to touch on these issues because the plight of the lonely ego is not assisted by our customary and conventional ideas. Our selves, carried as it were in the womb of various groups—race, culture, gender, et cetera—now find that all of these are only partial functions of the truly human. In being wholly contained in these partialities we cannot attain to the universality of being that is implied in the phrase 'true manhood'. Yet our self yearns for this.

I think that for most of us today the idea of mankind is limited to those men, women and children who are actually in existence now in this world. If mankind, or womankind for that matter, is to become a living reality for us then we must begin to envisage its origin, evolution and future development, not only physically but as a consciousness that has been evolving through the aeons and ages. Perhaps we shall even have to imagine that this reality—mankind, anthropos—is still undergoing its embryonic, foetal development, is in one sense only about to be born! The current Darwinian and neo- or post-Darwinian theories are inadequate; they seek to derive the human being from a dead cosmos. Older cosmogonies held a different view, seeing the cosmos as a supersensible, spiritual, divine organism or Being. As it matured, this living Being gradually condensed, stage by stage until, as with a human embryo, it manifested in a body perceptible to the senses and with even a bony skeleton—its mineral rocks. Later, we shall indicate how modern embryology offers a key to understand afresh these immensely significant, ancient, wisdom-filled cosmogonies within our modern consciousness.

The true organism 'mankind' must be an organism of free individuals. It is only today that we are becoming free in a real, not merely legal and democratic sense. As Socrates said, what most people mean by freedom is only to be the slaves of their lower natures and impulses. The free uniting of individuals in the light of this universal humanity is now needed for the healthy evolution of the human being quite apart from overcoming personal isolation. Only from each separate human being, and in full awareness of the whole being of humanity, can we go forward. The old sustaining foundational groupings must gradually be understood as *organs* of this great, universal and evolving humanity.

9. Materialism Grips Medicine

Vesalius's illustrated book of human anatomy was produced and published in 1543, the same year as Copernicus's book on the solar system was published posthumously. These two works signalled the arrival of a new, materialistic consciousness and an avalanche of natural-scientific work followed. In medicine this has led to the dominance of structured, spatial ideas (in other words, anatomical ideas), and the origin of disease was sought in structural change. To this day, the ultimate judgement on the cause of death is based on the post-mortem findings in the corpse. The causes of diseases are sought in the realms of micro-organisms and of chemical and physical entities. Scientific knowledge of diseases has become ever further removed from human experience. Two philosophic streams, parallel but distinct, lay at the origin of this. Descartes distinguished between the *res extensa* (material/mechanical) and the *res logicans* (immaterial/involving consciousness). Locke distinguished primary and secondary qualities. He gave to weight, extension, shape, motion, touch, the status of primary qualities and to colour, smell, taste, tone, the status of secondary qualities, signifying that they were not objectively real in the object perceived but arose only subjectively through the different senses in man. He thus gave to touch the unique honour of being real whereas to the other senses he gave mere subjective status, not outwardly belonging to the object but only inwardly to the perceiving subject. (When someone is not sure whether he is awake or dreaming he pinches himself to make sure!) In this way exclusive materialism, touchability, became the 'touchstone' of scientific reality and explanation.

So this has been the dominant current of modern medicine. But there has been a very different line as well. Looking back to ancient times we find that medicine was mostly bound up with the temple and it was in Greece that there began a separation of secular from religious medicine. In legend, Hippocrates walked out of the temple leaving his book behind as a farewell offering, and it has become customary to trace clinical, observational medicine from that time. However, apart from this Hippocratic stream of thinking, the temple medicine centred in Epidauros and other great sites continued to flourish. Here, treatment was on psychological grounds and inner soul-development was the means. Such treatment, culminating in the vision of the god Asclepius beheld during the temple sleep, must have been nearer to the experience of initiation in the mystery centres than to a visit to a Hippocratic physician. The two streams of medicine were on friendly terms with each other and it seems that the secular stream, together with Aristotle's science and his vast knowledge of herbs, was eventually expelled from Greece by the Emperor Justinian and went east beyond the Persian Gulf to Gondishapur and then Baghdad. From there it came back to the West with the spread of Islam to Spain, Sicily and Europe. This knowledge contributed enormously to the growth of medical knowledge in Renaissance Europe. The temple/mystery stream, on the other hand, seems mostly to have gone underground. A relic remained in Church circles as the practice of exorcism where a priest, having diagnosed that the patient was demonically possessed, battled with the devil using certain cultic practices. Records of similar practices have been found all over the world, and some continue to this day.

A sort of turning-point came towards the end of the eighteenth century when the exorcism practised by Gassner, a Roman Catholic priest and famous Healer of Württenburg, was confronted by the secular physician Mesmer who proceeded to bring about similar phenomena by what he called animal magnetism. During the nineteenth century such phenomena underwent cycles of popularity and contempt. What was sometimes called magnetism became known as mesmerism and then hypnotism. Somnambulistic states were studied and behaviour which would medically be called 'hysterical' contributed to and confused the observations and attempted explanations. What was really going on? The natural-scientific movement had established its foundations firmly in the physical sciences. Chemistry had now emerged from alchemy in a way that purged substance of all its qualitative aspects (these aspects which were to feature strongly later in Jung's explorations). Meanwhile, biology was mastered by Darwinism. It came to be felt that it was possible for everything to be grasped and understood by ordinary sense- and brain-bound intellect. However, the soul continued to cause trouble by producing all the hysterical phenomena that were then experimentally studied by Mesmer and his successors. Such phenomena have always been familiar to 'medicine men', shamans and their like, but these men had had to go through a deep and soul-changing training, an initiation process, before they could cope with these riddles. Now the prevailing science sought to include the profundity of this realm also in its empire and make it subject only to all-conquering logic and intellect, leaving no room for wonder, mystery or freedom. So it was that, through many successors to Mesmer down to the Parisian psychiatrist Pierre Janet and the aforementioned Charcot, the scientific approach to the soul proceeded, culminating with the work of Sigmund Freud. Now the unaided intellect could unravel the mysteries of dreams and the genius of art and religion, explaining them in such terms as the Oedipus complex: every man wants to murder his father and sleep with his mother. Had sex now replaced God?

As the nineteenth century came to an end after four hundred years of natural-scientific endeavour—a spiritual endeavour by individual scientists of immense and perhaps unparalleled intensity—what riches were there that could be bequeathed to the twentieth century? Firstly, an enormous accumulation of observations and attempts to order and clarify them. Never before had there been such study of the physical, sensory phenomena of the world experimentally verified.

In the medical field, more and more individually distinguished diseases were identified and named, resulting in an ever-increasing need for specialists. There had also been introduced the beginnings of vaccination and immunization. Vaccination against smallpox was first introduced from Turkey towards the end of the eighteenth century but only became widespread after 1796 when Edward Jenner began to use a cowpox vaccine against this almost universal plague. Immunity precautions and treatment of tetanus and diphtheria were then started before 1900. This early work has led to the huge explosion of knowledge about and research into the complexities of the so-called immune processes. All this work proceeds on the basis of purely chemical, molecular concepts, and has as its ideal the complete elimination of various diseases as may have happened in the case of smallpox. It is a genocidal idea carried over from warfare into medicine, and one which seems to me to rule today's medicine.

The nineteenth century saw immense developments in chemistry and physics, atomic theory came to dominate chemistry and the division between so-called organic and inorganic chemistry broke down with the laboratory synthesis of urea. This also led to the demise of vitalistic ideas that held living nature to be the expression of a special vital force. At the same time, ideas of evolution had been put forward by many scientists and thinkers. The French biologist Lamarck, who died in 1829, and Erasmus Darwin (the grandfather of Charles Darwin) put forward views on the evolution of species in opposition to the previous doctrine of Linnaeus of the immutability of species. (Goethe's views on metamorphosis of plants are often put forward as related to these views but his whole way of seeing and thinking the phenomena of nature really go beyond any of these theories.) Oken was also a significant figure who, by 1810, had already stated that the embryo in its development recapitulates the ancestral stages. Another very important contributor was Robert Chambers who was a lawyer by profession but whose work *Vestiges of Creation* (1844) received most of the angry rejection from traditionalists and churchmen, the upholders of the biblical tradition of creationism, which left the field comparatively clear for Charles Darwin, whose work carried the day. Natural selection and survival of the fittest were put forward as the causes of evolution and made God and creationism unnecessary. Natural forces could now account for the upward evolution of species as recorded in geological records, and at the top emerged the human being. In this way it came about that the human being is, for science, merely the highest animal and nothing more. Of those three realms, God, man and Nature, or the Infinite, the indefinite and the finite, only Nature—the realm of the finite—has remained as a significant and useful area of study.

The immense triumphs of science have been in the conquest of Nature from the realms of the atomic and subatomic to those of molecular biology. The finite implies a beginning and ending, a limitation in time as well as in space. Astrophysics has been obsessed with the idea of the origin of the cosmos in the Big Bang. An end of the cosmos in the so-called 'universal heat death' has long been accepted as a consequence of the second law of thermodynamics, which introduced direction into the laws of physics which hitherto could run both forwards and backwards equally. The question always arises as to what pre-existed the Big Bang, and a similar question has arisen in regard to the individual human being. Did he pre-exist the big bang of conception or, as has been maintained in the Western world since Aristotle, was he really a new creation? Should we dismiss Virgil's account of how Aeneas, on his journey through the underworld, met souls awaiting their next incarnations?

It has been a dogma of natural science that physics is the fundamental science and that other sciences must be based on and reduced to physics. In spite of the word 'physics' in its Greek origin being the name for living nature, it has come to mean the science of the inorganic. I think that the time has arrived when we must re-establish biology as the fundamental science and see physics as the science of the corpse of the living. The problem should be as to how dead matter and the mineral originated out of a pre-existent living organism, rather than of how life originated out of dead matter. I think it was Nietzsche who pointed to the oyster and asked which came first, the oyster or the shell. It is possible that the present interest in chaos theory is a symptom of the need to establish the realm of the indefinite distinct from the finite and infinite. It must however be clarified that, according to the way Fabre d'Olivet developed the theme, the realm of the indefinite is the realm of human free will as distinct from destiny, which belongs to the realm of the finite, and Providence, which belongs to the realm of the infinite.

It will need great courage and a great cooperative effort to reinterpret the factual findings of biology and anthropology so as to reveal the full relationship of man, animal and the other kingdoms of Nature. At present the doctrine of the human being as higher animal is so entrenched that it impedes the development of insights into the nature of human illness and of healing. It inhibits the affirmation of the spiritual meaning of human evolution and is leading to the pandemic of world-wide mental depression predicted by the World Health Organization, and already foreseen by, for example, Alexis Carrel in his book *Man the Unknown* in 1935.

10. Evolution—Facts, Theories and Myths

Now we must distinguish between an enormous, wonderful, discovery and accumulation of facts and the speculative theories that attempt to order and explain them. This is not easy as the two have become so entwined. Maybe what needs to be done is to stand the theories on their heads or turn them inside out. It is still a question as to whether the older cosmologies, deriving this world by stages from a purely spiritual origin of a multitude of supersensible beings rather than from matter, were not better than our materialistic modern theories. Of course, these old cosmologies with their majesty, depth and wondrous insights were couched in mythological forms and they appealed to a consciousness long vanished, a much more dreamlike and even clairvoyant consciousness. Through the discipline of six hundred years of developing scientific thinking we have now established a standard, a criterion to be met by our knowledge in all its branches; it must be achieved in full waking consciousness and no longer with vestiges of the old dreamlike mysticisms. This is one aspect of the challenge that Steiner took up in presenting again and again from many different points of view his cosmological and evolutionary spiritual science. He maintained and demonstrated that today human beings can achieve an inner soul development that extends their perception beyond sense perception to the regions of the spirit. Ancient primordial human wisdom had come to early mankind in the form of revelation. It was reborn in the achievement of Steiner as spiritual science, the science of the spirit; it had undergone the necessary metamorphosis brought

about by the Christian revelation of a spirit reality for each
individual ego.

The philosopher Schopenhauer made the suggestion that
it was the unborn child that first brought the future parents
together. One could say that the unborn child first incarnated into the warmth engendered in the love between the
parents. Steiner looked back in cosmic memory to a very
early planetary form of the Earth, and noted that this form
extended only as far as the element of Fire, or warmth. The
'idea' of the human being was also then present, but
embodied only as something we could describe as 'organized
warmth'. Perhaps one can see Schopenhauer's suggestion as
a recapitulation of this cosmic origin of man and earth?

Steiner was able to describe further incarnations of the
Earth. A second planetary embodiment proceeded as far as
the element of Air. As in the Greek Pneuma, Air was not just
a semi-material element but soul, spirit. Taking further the
idea of recapitulation by the incarnating soul, after the initial
warmth that united the parents is it not a communion of
soul, a mutuality of breathing, that holds them together? A
third embodiment of the Earth descended as far as the Water
element. As the Air element leads us to the region of the
soul, so the watery element now becomes a gateway to life. A
real mixing of the living fluid elements comes about. Only at
the fourth embodiment does our planetary development
proceed to a solid element, Earth, and to separateness of
existence. The soul enters gradually into the embryo which
only gradually hardens into solid elements. At the first stages
in embryological development it is the membranes that will
surround the future embryo that are developed. It is the
environment into which the child can enter that is first
established and only then does the embryo itself appear and

begin its own growth and development. As König, Poppelbaum and Weihs have shown, this development recapitulates
the Earth's own development. In Poppelbaum's words 'The
development of the human embryonic sheaths and appen-
dages is a reproduction of cosmic events in a material
medium'. In a somewhat comparable manner, Jaworski saw
the moon as earth's placenta. The embryo and foetus see
only one side of the placenta and we see only one side of the
moon, which reflects or mediates the sun and the whole
cosmos to us as the placenta mediates the maternal cosmos
to the foetus. (The placenta has long been invested with
profound symbolism. Margaret Murray, the Egyptologist,
drew attention to the custom in ancient Egypt of carrying the
Pharaoh's placenta like a banner in his processions. This
custom, she pointed out, was the origin of the national flag.)
   In Greek mythology we find an initial period of chaos
which signifies emptiness:

In the beginning of Things, black-winged Night
Into the bosom of Erebos dark and deep
Laid a wind-born egg, and as the seasons rolled,
Forth sprang Love, gleaming with wings of gold.
Like to the whirlings of wind, Love the Delight—
And Love with Chaos in Tartaros laid him to sleep;
And we, his children, nestled, fluttering there,
Till he led us forth to the light of the upper air.

Aristophanes

Here we can discern an echo of that primordial origin out of
chaos, emptiness and darkness in which only the warmth of
love manifested. Steiner describes the birth of Earth history
as incorporating successive periods of recapitulation of the
earlier planetary embodiments beginning with a state of

embodiment which reached only to the realm of warmth. This period he called the Polarian epoch, and many mythologies encapsulate this time in the image of the World Egg. From the action of this warmth of love arose the mythological upper and lower eggshell: Heaven and Earth, or Ouranos and Gaia. Ouranos lay on Gaia every night and she bore the twelve Titans and Titanesses. In his book *The Gospel of Hellas*, Frederick Hiebel recalled that the number twelve was always connected with the appearance of space, and we see an indication in the myth that to the germinal condition of warmth, light and air (and therefore space) were added. This development was the epoch of Earth history that Steiner called Hyperborea.

The youngest of the Titans, Kronos, rebelled and with his wife Rhea assumed government. They had six children: Poseidon, Hades, Zeus, Demeter, Hestia, Hera, so that, with the parental unit, the number seven prevailed, a number traditionally connected with rhythm and time. We have now entered the phase of Earth's development where the gaseous condition is densifying to the more rhythm-permeated fluid condition, the epoch that Steiner called Lemuria, whose geological echo we know today as the Mesozoic period, the time of the great reptiles.

In due course Kronos was himself dethroned by Zeus and the age of the Olympian gods and goddesses commenced. This was the age generally known as Atlantis, the memory of which was recorded by Plato, and which is now known to geology as the Tertiary period. During this time the condition of the earth was slowly increasing in density.

This Atlantean period ended with the great Flood when Noah entered into the Ark, whose measurements are said to have had the same proportions as the human body. Jaworski, amongst others, has seen a correspondence between the Flood and our human birth amidst the flood of amniotic fluid. So we could see Atlantis as picturing the period of the foetal development of man, or our foetal life in the womb as the recapitulation of Atlantis. (The earlier Lemurian age is also recapitulated in the preceding embryonic development.) Geologically the time of the Flood corresponds with the last Ice Age and Jaworski related the recurrent Ice Ages to the birth pangs of Mother Earth, the 'Geon'.

This leads to the question as to when did what we may call mankind originate, granting that the human being became really *born* only at the end of Atlantis. Further, what is the relation between the human and the animal? Jaworski's Geon, the living organism of the earth, must have given birth to the animals over long, long periods of time but they were born prematurely, so to speak. We have become accustomed to the picture of the so-called biological tree, in which the supposed evolutionary process grew up the trunk passing from unicellular creatures of bewildering variety to more complex creatures consisting of colonies of cells differentiated in form and function. In this way arose branches from the trunk such as the multitude of the invertebrates, creatures without backbones: the polyps, in which an inside and outside occur, sponges, starfish and their metamorphosis into sea-urchins. The starfishes are formed as pentagons, like the human vertebrae, and the sea urchin is globular like the human skull. Then there are the vast and contrasting worlds of the worms and the molluscs, where the worms develop segmentation and the molluscs, for example snails and slugs, shellfish and octopuses, all remain unsegmented. As a sort of culmination of the invertebrates are the insects, lobsters and crabs, with their external skeletons, segmentation and articulated limbs. Now comes the great transition to the realm of the vertebrates. Many interesting theories have been put forward to elucidate this profound metamorphosis. One of the most suggestive was expressed by the great physiologist-biologist Gaskell in his book *The Origin of Vertebrates*. There he seeks to demonstrate that in the lamprey, a primitive fish with a vertebral backbone, its larval form shows an invertebrate form kindred to the limulus, the king crab. In this creature, as with all articulata, such as insects, crustacea, etc., the nervous chain runs along *below* the intestinal canal whereas in the vertebrates the nervous system lies above the intestine. In so far as the nervous system is very connected with the important sensory organ of the skin, it can be considered as an 'outer' part of the organism. The intestine, on the other hand, is very much 'inner'. Now Gaskell saw how the nervous system of the invertebrate grew and grew, so to speak, until it encircled and enclosed the intestine within itself. The alimentary, intestinal organ was incorporated into the nervous system as the central canal within the spinal cord. The inner became the outer. Now a new alimentary system becomes necessary and this is formed by an interiorization, an inturning or infolding of the skin of the lower side. The outer has become inner! Gaskell demonstrated this in some detail in the embryology of the lamprey; could his work encourage us to participate more imaginatively in the elucidation of many other metamorphoses?

The biological tree proceeded by way of the fishes and the amphibians, frogs, toads, etc, then reptiles to birds and the marsupials and mammals. These last with hot blood were the true animals for the Greeks, the 'Theria'. At the top of the tree appeared the human being. Along the trunk were supposed to be primitive animal forms from which grew out the branches with the forms we have mentioned. The fossil remains, which have constituted a main 'proof' of this thesis, have had to be moved more and more to the tips of the branches, leaving the trunk and branches to be filled with the missing links. The essence of this picture, as it has come to dominate our current views of the nature of the human being, is that the whole tree, apart from the topmost tips, represents animal evolution. Because of this, the topmost tips have also come to be regarded as merely animal. All this happened through the concept of the survival of the fittest. 'Fit for what?' we may ask. The answer is disturbingly taut-ological: Fit to survive in the battle for survival! When we look at the myriad forms in their uncountable variety it looks more as if *all* variations naturally occurring were naturally selected, instead of just the so-called 'best'.

Against this picture Jaworski proposed that the central trunk of this tree represented the embryological develop-ment of the human being throughout its whole growth. He therefore saw mankind as the earliest of all the creatures, although, as in the embryo, of so soft a substance that no fossil record would exist. As the embryo of mankind devel-oped its internal organs, so—outwardly exteriorized in the branches—came about the organisms, all the different classes in the animal kingdom. The phyla, the great groups of creatures within the animal kingdom are the human being's organs exteriorized. We could also say that the animal kingdom is the analysis, the human is the synthesis. The human being is not just a higher animal but rather the synthesis of all the creatures in the animal world. Jaworski was not a mystic but a physician and biologist who was driven to these perceptions by long study and contemplations. His views serve to corroborate most fittingly many of Steiner's conclusions drawn from the sources of his spiritual science.

This view of evolution and the biological tree also draws our attention to the slowness of human evolution. According to Steiner, the human being was the first to be conceived but the last to be truly born. When Noah stepped out of the Ark on Mount Ararat a rainbow manifested for the first time, for until then the atmosphere had been water and air mixed in a way that it was not possible for a rainbow to form. After the Flood, the air cleared and human beings began to breathe properly for the first time; it could now be said that the human being was *born*. In contrast the animals had all been prematurely born; they were not able to hold back but descended into dense incarnation whilst the human being was held back in a more ethereal body. With this descent the animal kingdom became confined in bodies that were very specialized instruments. The human being, however, has remained omnipotential, with the possibility of inventing all the tools and capacities which, as organs, imprison animals in one-sided specialism. People invent knives, forks, etc. which the lion's claws and teeth have become, but they can also invent oars to row a boat and wings of aeroplanes to fly in the air. The wasp makes paper to build its nest and cannot but do so; people have discovered how to manufacture paper and can do so or not as they choose. All our clevernesses were incorporated earlier into the very bodies of different animals.

So, we find that whilst the human being has retained its omnipotentiality by remaining closest to the embryonic form, the animals have diverged increasingly from this archetype. Jaworski saw the animals as representing human organs, tissues and cells analysed into their distinctive groups. He found that the human form includes all the divergent animal forms within, synthesized, just as Noah's Ark contained all the animals. Jaworski was perplexed for a time by the tortoises, which are reptiles like the snakes yet almost spherical instead of almost endlessly elongated. Then he saw them as livers with the carapace of the diaphragm overlying them. The colours of the bile even find themselves in the colours of the tortoiseshell. The human liver has, amidst its thousands of chemical functions, a polarity between the glucose-glycogen metabolism and the bile. The sugar polarity finds itself outside in the bees and the honeycomb, hexagonal as the liver is in its inner structure. The tortoises are very long-lived and full of vitality, slow but obsessionally fixed in their determined direction. What a contrast to the busy bees! The liver, as its name implies, is full of life and it can still regrow even if over a half has been removed. When Prometheus, whose name signifies foresight, was nailed upon the rocky crags of the Caucasus, an eagle, the bird of Zeus, came every day and tore out his liver. Every day our own livers are broken down by catabolic processes and every night are rebuilt by the sweet anabolic ones. Zeus represents the fully conscious forces of the head which arise on the destructive catabolic processes. Consciousness itself pushes the anabolic processes down into the liver, the natural home for all clairvoyant, prophetic forces, and keeps them imprisoned there, asleep in the unconscious. The benevolent centaur Cheiron, who was able to teach the arts of healing to Asclepius because of his atavistic Atlantean clairvoyance, was the one who eventually set Prometheus free. Prometheus could only be saved from being cast into Tartarus, the abode of the wicked in Hades, if a substitute for him could be found. Cheiron volunteered because, owing to an unfortunate mistake, he had already suffered an immortal, unhealable wound at the hands of Heracles. Prometheus—the new future clairvoyance—needed the sacrifice of the old instinctive clairvoyance.

The Roman god Jupiter is said to rule over the liver and over the wise judgement of the head. Does not the tortoise also remind one of the skull arching over the soft matter within? Further, the tortoise has a unique anatomical feature. It has its shoulder girdle inside its rib cage. How did it get there? König demonstrated how the human body is metamorphosed into the head. In the foetus the body is bent forwards in the embryonic posture. In life it becomes upright and after death, according to König, the forces of the body are folded over backwards, as it were, and become the head of the next incarnation. Following König's scheme, we find that the body is turned backwards into the form of the head in such a way that the shoulder blades become the sphenoid bones, now inside the metamorphosed rib cage which has become cranium. Steiner's indications tell us that our head comes from a previous incarnation and, in contrast, our liver, as centre of the metabolism and therefore of our human forces of will, points to the future. This connection between the tortoise and the head takes on an ironic twist in the following postscript to the Prometheus story.

The story of Prometheus was composed into a Trilogy by Aeschylus, of which only one part survives. Aeschylus had to flee from Athens, accused of betraying the secrets of the mysteries. He went to Sicily in Magna Graecia and as he walked one day, so the legend records, an eagle with a tortoise in its claws flew over. It dropped the tortoise on the head of Aeschylus and killed him!

So the head can be seen as a synthesis of the body, whose

limbs function in the head as the jaws. All the animals that can be 'found' in the organs of the body are also in the head. The birds that Jaworski saw in the lungs and chest are there in the head as the soaring philosophic thoughts of the eagle (the symbol of St John, author of the fourth Gospel in the New Testament), the chattering of the sparrows, the lovely lyrical thoughts of the swallows and so on. The head mirrors the body; in the head we 'reflect' on something and in the head the body is reversed into mirror-image, left side of the body in the right brain and vice versa.

The uterus also has an interesting link with one aspect of the head. The brain lies in the cavity of the skull very much as the foetus in the uterus. Now a woman's reproductive cycle follows a moon rhythm and the brain—like the moon—reflects; we conceive thoughts in our heads but our thoughts are only reflections of reality. In the uterus, however, real physical reproduction occurs and real babies are conceived. Every planet has traditionally been connected with a metal and silver is the metal of the moon. Silver makes the best mirror and silver salts are used in photographic reproduction. In Greek mythology the moon goddess Artemis occurs in two forms: on mainland Greece Artemis was a young maiden huntress and midwife to animals whereas in Ephesus she was the mature goddess of wisdom. Do they, perhaps, correspond to the waxing and waning moon and to reproduction and contemplative reflection?

The metamorphosis of the body into the head is a metamorphosis in time, not just in space. It is a metamorphosis, as Steiner indicated, from one incarnation into another, perhaps after centuries. Once we have become able to envisage metamorphosis over extended time spans we may look for it in areas closer to our experience. Poppelbaum studied the common earthworm and its similarity to a caterpillar and was led to ask why it did not also metamorphose into a butterfly. It is only in the imago stage, as butterfly, that the caterpillar can reproduce. Poppelbaum sees the earthworm as able to reproduce in a permanent larval stage, so what has become of the forces with which it would have metamorphosed into a butterfly? He makes the revealing suggestion that with these forces the earthworm helps to fertilize the earth, as it were sacrificing its further development and giving its unused forces to the earth. Another area offers us a different type of example. When a baby is born its body is by no means finished. Its limbs, for example, are still very unformed and its face still undeveloped. The brain has to be organized gradually, the immune system is scarcely active, the first teeth have not yet erupted and other organs are still only coming into their proper functions. During the first seven years of life, until approximately the change of teeth, the child is mostly absorbed in the task of building its future body. Its inherited body is a sort of model on which to base its building activity. The individuality coming into this 'architect's drawing', as it were, may slavishly copy this drawing with its inherited gifts and defects or it may be strong enough to overcome these and to some extent create its own individual body. At seven years of age, according to Steiner, some of the forces used in this building activity become surplus to the requirements of the organic function and available for metamorphosis into the forces of memory and thinking. Today, under the pressure of intellectual education, this metamorphosis may be prematurely accelerated, leaving the body inadequately transformed. In this way the ground may well be prepared for illness in later life.

We have been suggesting that because the human being

remains nearer to its foetal form, in other words remains less evolved rather than becoming more evolved in its bodily form, forces that have been utilized in the animal for specialization have been transformed in the human being into mental capacities. We have developed our capacity to invent and to think by remaining less adapted to one-sided specialized environments, by remaining more childlike.

11. *The Single and the Whole*

There are two aspects to the situation in which human beings find themselves at this stage of evolution, and both present us with crises and questions. One aspect is the need to become a whole single human individual. Ordinarily, the first half of life is concerned with entering into and mastering some aspect of our world, the world of bits and pieces, and the second half of life is about growing again into the heavenly or spiritual world, the world of wholes. Wholes are beings, and as such produce effects. Some wholes, for example persons, are apparent to the senses, but most of the world of wholes are supersensible. For an age nurtured in natural science and its insistence on sense-perceptibility this affords immense difficulties. On a simple level the problems arose in the famous conversation between Goethe and Schiller. Goethe sketched his imagination of the *Urpflanze*, the wholeness of plant which gives rise to all the parts of the plant and all the varieties and species of plants. Schiller responded by affirming that this was an idea not a perception. To this the aggrieved Goethe retorted with the comment that as he could *see* his Idea *with his eyes* he was, understandably, very pleased about it! In ancient times the world of spiritual beings, innumerable in grades and types, was perceptible to people. In our own time, although many people in many parts of the world can still see as far as the land of the Little People, with our ever-deepening incarnation into the physical body most of us have progressively lost these ancient faculties and an abyss has opened between this world and the other. We do cross this threshold when we go to sleep but we also lose consciousness and cannot remember our sleep experiences. The particular chaos and crisis of the twentieth century and beyond owes a lot to the fact that mankind in general has actually crossed this threshold, that is to say, we are now interacting with spiritual beings in our waking life but are aware of it only on an unconscious level. We continue to use ideas and concepts of the physical world when in reality we are trying to interact with the spiritual world. We are blind to the very world in which we try to find our way, and the challenge for us is to wake up to these new realities in which we live our lives.

The second aspect of our situation has arisen, as polar opposite to the first, in the form of the global economy. The world has become one and we can no longer handle problems in isolation from each other. Regional and national issues have to be grasped and handled not in relation to the individual but in relation to the whole world. It is obvious in regard to economics and it is becoming more and more clear that even health matters cannot be managed locally however immense the differences are that exist from one region to another. But the question now arises whether it is enough to approach the oneness of our world through technology. How much understanding can this approach alone give us?

Let us look at the idea of humanity as an organism. We usually think of an organism as a physical unity, all its component cells belonging together and in physical connection. Now consider a flock of birds. Do not the individual birds act in unison with each other, taking off, wheeling in the air and so on as one 'organism'? Even more so does a beehive or ant colony act as a single organism, although to our outer observation it consists of a multitude of separate organisms. Many observations have been made showing that what happens to a creature in one part of the world is immediately sensed by its relatives across the globe. Rupert Sheldrake has drawn powerful attention to such facts. They seem to point to a realm which C.G. Jung, from another side, was compelled to envisage and investigate, that of the 'collective unconscious'. Is the human race, then, an organism composed of the multitude of individuals? Jung was forced to accept that below the individual unconscious consisting of forgotten personal experiences there are deeper levels in which ancestral and racial memories lie buried and forgotten. Henri Bergson, in his study *Matter and Memory* at the beginning of the twentieth century, demonstrated that the phenomena of memory could not be explained out of physiology. Memory is revealed as not just physically contained but as passing across generations and millennia. It is supersensory.

As early as 1911 Henry Bernard drew attention to the importance of colony formation in evolution. Successive waves or levels of colony formation are revealed in the evolutionary process. Colony formation necessitates cooperation, not competition between the separate cells. We human beings have now reached the evolutionary crisis where the individual units, the separate persons of our common whole, are becoming free individuals. We are actually maturing *out* of Nature, out of being contained within families, nations, races. In such groups, humanity was still really within Nature, as a lion is within its 'group soul'. Only today more and more individuals are becoming isolated and potentially free individuals, that is to say in reality a whole person, rather than an Englishman or an Asian, a man or a woman and so on. The content of such a person needs to be truly human, with a humanity embodying its whole past, present and future. We can recall the saying of Lao Tse:

He, who being a man remains a woman, will become a universal channel. As a universal channel the eternal virtue will never forsake him. He will become a child again.

Auguste Comte was amongst the first to proclaim in scientific-philosophic terms the idea of mankind as *Le Grand Être*, a living Being. The Russian philosopher Soloviev wrote of Comte:

It is still greater merit and glory of Comte's that he indicated more clearly, fully and decisively than any of his predecessors that 'something' other—the collective whole which, in its inner essence and not merely externally, surpasses every individual man and actually completes him, both ideally and really: he indicated 'humanity' as a living positive unity embracing us, as pre-eminently 'The Great Being', 'Le Grand Être'.

Soloviev saw Comte's Grand Être—Humanity—as God the Holy Spirit beginning to incarnate into the organism of free persons, humankind risen out of nature. H.G. Wells in his book *God the Invisible King* was approaching the same idea.

An organism is not only differentiated spatially into its systems, organs, tissues, but also in time. To grasp the reality of an organism it is not enough to dissect and anatomize it, we must also move towards imagining its wholeness in time, its life from birth to death grasped as inwardly differentiated in developing ages. Did not Shakespeare indicate this in his well-known words:

All the world's a stage,
And all the men and women merely players:
They have their exits and their entrances;

And one man in his time plays many parts,
His acts being seven ages.

We cannot grasp this temporal whole with our senses, they can only give us the momentary cross-section in space, a sort of inert relic. It is possible, however, that we can follow Goethe and develop a faculty of Imagination which would enable us to grasp 'Ideas' that are in time as well as space.

As physical beings we cannot say we are whole. Since the division into sexes, mythically with Adam and Eve, evolutionarily probably in the Mesozoic times, we are only half a true human being. Steiner pointed out that in Genesis the first creation of man should be translated as 'male-female created he him' not male *and* female. In our time the psychologist C.G. Jung saw that any endeavour to become a full person must include the redeeming of the lost other sex in us. Men must endeavour to help the female in the soul, the anima, to mature and become reintegrated into the conscious personality. And women must bring forward their male aspect, the animus, to join equally with their female persona. The offspring of such male/female unions would now make it possible for us to understand the quotation from Lao-Tse that I gave earlier, and regain the vision of Georg Groddeck who saw the human archetype as Male, Female and Child, a trinity rather than a duality. Christianity, also, contains the saying 'Unless you become again as little children, you shall in no way enter into the kingdom of heaven'.

In our psyches also we find we are only potentially one and whole. We all harbour within us a shadow-side which we do not perceive and acknowledge, though our friends and enemies invariably do! Oscar Wilde portrayed such a figure in *The Picture of Dorian Gray* and R.L. Stevenson did so in *The*

Strange Case of Dr Jekyll and Mr Hyde. In every serious discipline aimed at developing the individuality, the confrontation with and integration of this *doppelgänger,* shadow or 'double', is of the greatest importance. It can open the door to the other side of the personality which ordinarily lies in the so-called unconscious, in the oblivion of forgetfulness. Let us remember that von Hartmann affirms that what is called the unconscious could as well be called the super- or supra-conscious. Everyone belongs to two worlds, and our time is compelling or urging us to open and expand our consciousness to embrace not only this world but also the other, the forgotten half of our existence, the spiritual world.

12. Finding Our Way Through the Underworld

The living cosmos of the ancient world contrasts starkly with today's impression of the universe as vast, purely physical, and probably dead. Immense efforts are being made to find some spark of life somewhere in the heavenly bodies. At the same time we are mapping the human genome, seeking to make of our living organism a mere physical, chemical machine. We praise the scientific efforts that have brought us many helpful technical triumphs in medicine and surgery, but we must also admit the loss of a sense of meaning and purpose in existence that brings increasing disorders of the soul.

If we look back to ancient Greece we find stories that can throw some light on our situation. The Greek heroes such as Herakles, Orpheus, Perseus had all to venture into the underworld, the world of the dead, which had become for the Greeks the world of 'the shades'. People were at that time so deeply identified with their physical bodies that at death they could only feel that the soul accompanied the body into the earth. Today we have, through our technical achievements, succeeded in bringing the forces of the underworld, in other words the sub-earthly forces of electricity and magnetism in particular, up and all around us. Modern people are all passing willy-nilly through the underworld!

Of the Greek heroes, Orpheus had successfully made the journey and recovered his lost soul Eurydice, but then he mistakenly looked back and lost her again. Virgil records the journey of Aeneas, accompanied by the Cumaean Sybil to visit his dead father and, centuries later, it was Virgil himself who became the guide of Dante through hell and purgatory. Modern Western societies, living as they do in an atmosphere increasingly full of radiations and electromagnetic forces, could certainly be seen as having crossed a threshold and as traversing this same journey through hell. We were led here by the Industrial Revolution, itself the fruit of scientific revolution and materialism, and are now experiencing the social and personal confusion it brings on many different levels. How difficult it is sometimes not to be a 'lost soul' in this self-created underworld! This is both a tragedy and a vital opportunity, for the way out and forward cannot be found by looking back as Orpheus did. To our modern consciousness with its abstractions and intellectuality, everything has turned into shades, poor ghosts of the full reality. If we look backwards, nostalgically maybe, to earlier societies and their traditions, hoping to find solace and solutions there, then our very souls, our Eurydices, may fade into dubious memories or the ghostly insubstantiality of mere ideas. A new Promethean courage is called for. Shadowy ideas must be revivified and the spiritually empty intellectualism pervading not only science but also most of modern culture must be brought through a resurrection to be imbued with new life. It is our task, the task of our own solitary selves, our most central egos, to find the courage to discover in ourselves the core of living reality.

What are the implications of the statement that mankind in general has crossed the threshold between the material world and the spiritual world? There are, of course, many thresholds to be crossed during life, culminating in the great threshold crossing at death. It has become commonly recognized today that in the so-called near-death experiences individuals often confront a panorama of the life, a tableau in which the events of the late life are beheld. It is therefore not unreasonable to consider that at real death this life tableau experience marks the entry into the other world. Now, through archaeology, anthropology and other studies, we have had exposed to our vision in all the different cultures in the world a whole panorama of the life of mankind expressing the range of evolving human experiences. We can today behold, even during life, this panorama of our past history and evolution, both personal and general. Shakespeare differentiated the seven stages of an individual's life, which only together constitute the person, and the life panorama that is today spread out for us over the whole world enables us to grasp the totality of our humanity differentiated in time, in evolution. If we meet people today who manifest characteristics belonging to earlier epochs (even back as far as the epochs of Atlantis and Lemuria), this will serve to wake us up to all the particular levels of our collective unconscious. I have not yet heard of anyone experiencing the near-death tableau who has been tempted to value one group of memories more than another, and in the same way we may learn in life to value each contribution that the world and our experience of it offers to our personal evolution. In this context, I do think that reincarnation implies that each of us has lived, or will live in each culture in the course of time. Only when all are taken together can these pictures of the past help us to aspire to a grasp of the whole past evolution of humanity. Without this we cannot reach a living experience of mankind, Le Grand Être, of Comte.

There have been some interesting observations made by Karl König, in an illuminating essay *Meditations on the Endo-*

crine Glands. These glands belong to the blood system and they pour their secretions into the blood. He indicates how these glands, essentially seven in number, are organized in three pairs of two and a central one. The pineal gland in the centre of the head is polarized with the gonads, ovaries or testicles. The pituitary gland is polarized with the adrenals, and the thyroid gland with the thymus. The centre is formed by the parathyroids. In ancient times the pineal was the so-called third eye, the eye of spiritual clairvoyance. Odysseus, in Sicily on his epic journey, encountered the giant Poly-themus with a third eye in his forehead. He blinded this with a pole. Odysseus was characterized by his cleverness, and the developing intellectual cleverness of pre-Christian Greek culture banished the old clairvoyance, together with its per-ception of the spiritual world from which humanity has descended. We made this descent into the material world of generation by means of the gonads, or sex glands, which are polar to the pineal. So we trace the polarity here from our origin in the spiritual world through the recurring cycles of generation to a recovery of spiritual clairvoyance in the dis-tant future. Only then will the pineal gland once again sound the keynote of the accomplished, fully awake, clairvoyance of men and women. Between birth from the spiritual and such a resurrection into the spiritual lie the many evolutionary epochs of humankind. In this context we see that it is the blood (which according to occult tradition is the physical instrument of the non-physical ego) that plays a key role. The endocrine glands are in a special relationship with the blood since their substances, which are excreted directly into the bloodstream, serve, as does the blood, the total integrity of the body and not just one particular part. The finely regu-lated processes of the glandular system as a whole reveal its intimate connection with the unfolding stream of time. The blood, therefore, because of its participation in the work of the endocrine glands, brings the ego of the individual into a significant relationship with time; in the immune system, the blood enables the ego to address the issue of self and non-self in terms of space.

As human beings we all carry within us, in our underworld of the unconscious, aspects of the past, present and future, and the qualities and functions of our endocrine orchestra are constant reminders of the temporal procession of evolutionary epochs. The gonads are our window into the legendary epoch of Lemuria where, according to Steiner, the division of the sexes occurred and human life became more bound to an earthly ground. At the other end of the scale lies the pineal gland, immature at present. But is the media tendency to think in *head*lines perhaps a forerunner of the time when our intuitive, consciously achieved thoughts can act magically, directly into our will? The function of the endocrine glands in our organism has always been to link and harmonize the immensity of different functions and processes of our body and to bring them into relation with the wisdom of the cosmos, the 'will of the gods'. Pondering on our life as a social being on the one hand and the life of our physical organism on the other, we cannot escape the questions that demand new answers relating to our origins and our goals.

13. A Way Forward

The natural-scientific work of the last four to five centuries has expanded our knowledge of disease enormously. But if we are convinced that the materialistic anatomical concept of mankind and its diseases is inadequate, what can we move on to? Can we find other ways of tackling the problems of illness and, at the same time, rebuild a world of meaning and significance in place of the chance-ridden, accident-prone universe of our current conventional viewpoints?

This interlude in human evolution, in which intellect has undergone unparalleled development, albeit at the expense of imagination, feelings and intuition, can only be seen as necessary. We must include in our ideas of evolution not only the growth and metamorphosis of bodily forms but of the form of consciousness itself or, we could say, of the soul itself as well. Maybe we too easily assume that our ancestors thought and felt as we do. In his book *How to Know Higher Worlds*, Steiner has demonstrated that there is a way for modern people to expand their intellect into what he called living Imagination and enter into 'time as organism'. Then, without losing clarity of consciousness, they would begin to perceive the living organisms in the world developing in *time*, as well as the static, physical matter. He could see the living reality of the vegetable kingdom as well as its mineral content.

Hahnemann's studies were considerably enhanced by his discovery of certain polarities. This imaginative line of thinking is sure to continue bearing fruit for the medicine of the future. Nietzsche introduced the idea of the polarity of the Apollonian and Dionysian streams into his study of Greek tragedy. He saw this polarity wide-ranging in the whole of culture; he saw in sculpture more the expression of the Apollonic and in music more of the Dionysiac. This polarity corresponds to ancient paths to the upper and lower gods respectively. Apollo spoke through the oracles, whereas the path to Dionysos was through the mysteries and into the inner depths of the journey through the underworld. In Greek medicine we find Apollo as the main god of healing (Asclepius was his son). He is portrayed in his statue at Olympia as holding the balance and bringing order into the chaotic turmoil of life. Calm and reason are keynotes. Apollo keeps himself slightly aloof, ordering from a distance, even bringing death by arrow from a distance. By contrast, Dionysos plunges into the turmoil, the wild dance of reality, aiming not at calm but at ecstatic union with God. The Greek temple-medicine, as at Epidauros which was in close union with the mysteries, brought healing through renewal of the inward life of soul. Nietzsche sought to show these two streams united in Greek tragedy, the Dionysiac chorus on the circular orchestra and the Apollonic gods and heroes on the stage above.

We can find this polarity again in our own organisms, within which the brain and senses pole is clearly Apollonic and in our awake state relates us to the outer world. It is in this waking consciousness that we develop our sense of individuality, of self as opposed to not-self, and it is within the Delphic oracle centre that we find the Apollonic command to 'Know thyself'. From this awake consciousness has developed the multitudinous discovery of facts and their classification into types, groups and so on. In medicine this shows itself in the ever-increasing description of new diseases—

diseases grasped intellectually as distinct 'entities'. Behind these separate diseases we look for their causes in micro-organisms or genetic sources. The description of these has also become almost infinite. The diseases, as such, have become almost distinct from the human experience of ill-ness, and the aim arises to *eliminate* these diseases—an aim now quite separate from the aim of healing. The one-sided stream of the sun god Apollo came to extreme expression in the study of anatomy and its extension right down to the structure of molecules and atoms. It is spatial and is focused on the visual sense. The once fully alive, sun-irradiated wis-dom of the Apollonic oracles gradually dried up into a twenty-first century structural mentality. Just as the goddess Natura died away (even at the flowering of the School of Chartres the philosophers had lamented that this once living goddess had vanished from their sight) into our prevailing mechanistic natural science, so the glorious and radiant Apollo withered into our modern intellectualism.

Nietzsche has distinguished an ancient dithyrambic music, embodied in the tragedies of Aeschylus, from the music of the later Euripidean tragedies, noting that it had already lost some of its rich vitality. It is the art form of music, belonging as it does to the ear and dance rather than to the sculptural statics of space, which is able to bring in the time experience. In music, movement in time becomes the reality and it is possible for us, through our experience of music, to feel ourselves reconnecting both with the origins and also with the goals of existence. In this way, music enables us to re-establish our relationship with the Whole. The polarity of eye and ear are simply an aspect of this polarity of static Apol-lonic and the dynamic Dionysiac. The Apollonic has come to expression in surgery and in a medicine that is inwardly dominated by surgical thinking. The Dionysiac has been trying to come to a renewal in the psychologies of the unconscious throughout the twentieth century. Is there a third divinity also involved in the healing experience to mediate between these poles?

I should like to mention here an idea that has fallen into disuse as modern medicine has progressed. In alchemy there were three principles, Sal (Salt), Mercury and Sulphur, and we can today relate these in the organism to the nervous system, the rhythmic system and the metabolic-limb system respectively. Mercury, the principle of the rhythmic system, was seen to mediate between the Sal and Sulphur poles, each of which could otherwise dominate and lead to disease. Rhythm permeates all three systems. Even the brain is affected by the rhythm of the breathing, and the metabolism plays up into the heart beat. The interplay of these rhythms was the sphere of healing. In ancient times Mercury was one of the gods of healing, and his caduceus—two snakes inter-twined up a staff—is still often used today as symbol of the healing art. Mercury was the Roman name for the Greek deity Hermes.

The Greeks renamed the Egyptian god Thoth, Hermes Trismegistos. Thoth was the legendary founder of Egyptian culture, its science and medicine. In the Christian inter-pretation he became the Archangel Raphael, the patron saint of medicine and the healing arts. The Greek god Hermes has been brilliantly illuminated by W.F. Otto and by Karl Kerenyi; I think that one can see a more Apollonian approach in Otto and a more Dionysian one in Kerenyi. However that may be, Hermes does stand intimately related to both Apollo and Dionysos. The mystery centre of Dionysos was shared with his brother Apollo, whose oracle was within this sanctuary at Delphi; for six months in the year Apollo went to Hyperborea, leaving Delphi to his brother. Thus, the two streams were united. The infant Dionysos is portrayed carried on the arm of Hermes in the famous statue from the school of Praxitiles. Hermes and Apollo (his brother) became lifelong friends after an initial tiff. Now Hermes is by nature a mediator, carrying messages from Zeus to earth and guiding the souls of the dead to the underworld. He is the protector of ambassadors between states and he brings good luck (or bad); all unexpected, chance events are due to him. He is also guardian of all those who, legally or illegally, redistribute goods across frontiers. (We have already suggested that disease can be looked at as a right function in a wrong place and that healing entails only a redistribution or reordering.) Hermes was also called the 'shepherd of the flocks' and older sources reveal strange statues, the Herms, with the head of Hermes and an erect phallus, standing on a square base. These often stood at the thresholds of houses, cities, and at crossroads. One might even ask whether Hermes did not originate even earlier in the figure of Hermaphroditos: Hermes and his sister, Aphrodite the goddess of love, still united in androgynous form before the separation of the sexes. These Greek gods are imaginative images, archetypes, real forces active in the subconscious realms of the human psyche, actually experienced in those days in a dreamlike imaginative consciousness. With the gradual loss of this old clairvoyant faculty, decadence crept into the mysteries, and the world of the gods became a mere tradition and not any more a living experience. The Twilight of the Gods descended.

Their stories, however, like the parables of the Bible, challenge us with their imagery to unfold new ways of understanding the problems, both social and medical, that people suffer today. It was Paracelsus who emphasized that disease was not just an evil to be eliminated, but an opportunity for the sufferer to progress in spiritual development with Christ's help. In earlier Christian centuries there had been arguments as to whether the Greek god Asclepius or Christ was the true God of Healing. Healing as a divine power is very far from the medical consciousness of today.

14. Loss and Gain

To the physical world belongs the separateness of things, and the losing of the vision of a spiritual world filled with its multitudes of beings was for mankind like a descent from heaven. People found a world where they could gradually gain a sense of their individual existence, where they could discover their selves. From this time on death became a problem. One can follow this development in the course of Greek culture and also in the introduction of the historical perspective in ancient Hebrew culture, as Andrew Welburn has so well shown.

The old world, in which people had felt themselves off-spring of the living goddess Natura, died to them. 'Great Pan is dead,' was the cry in Plutarch's *On the Cessation of Oracles*. In this old world, people belonged through Nature to the whole living cosmos. How were they to survive into a time when the worlds of Nature and of the cosmos would be grasped only in abstract terms as just huge machines?

If people gained their individuality through this descent into the world of matter, of hate-divided things and of death, then with it they gained the possibility of freedom as individuals. To approach the realm of death means to place a foot on a very important threshold, and I think that we have seen enough indications in modern society to suggest that, for the most part, mankind has now crossed this threshold. As a consequence, thinking, feeling and will are now separating, just as science, art and religion have moved from a historical union to the modern position of separation and autonomy, within which, some say, they decline ever more into chaos.

Only a strengthened ego, the essentially human element in us and not to be confused with egotism, can help to bring order out of the chaos. It has become obvious, within the medical world, that not only has this chaos invaded the world of the patients but also that of the medical profession. It used to be that trust in the individual doctor was the most important part of healing. Now that scientific 'objectivity' has invaded the realm of therapy and has invented the self-styled double-blind trial as the only way of assessing treatment, the roles of both the individual doctor and the individual patient are eliminated from the observations. The only human elements in these assessments are removed. The personality of the individual doctor has to be negated so that objective facts can be studied, undisturbed by tiresome aspects of the soul such as wishes and persuasion and the deeper currents in the so-called transference relationship.

Georg Groddeck courageously pioneered, in the first third of the twentieth century, 'psychological' treatment of organic disease. Most of his patients were suffering from so-called incurable diseases, yet again and again he was able to change these illnesses radically for the better or completely to cure them. The future may well demand that the education of physicians will include adequate self-development to deepen the personality enough to deal with the prejudices, hang-ups and limitations of human understanding that are attendant on our prevailing materialistic, technological training.

And when the mind is quick'ned, out of doubt,
The organs, though defunct and dead before,
Break up their drowsy grave and newly move
With casted slough, and fresh legerity.
Shakespeare, *King Henry V* (Act IV, Scene i)

Today, doubt and self-doubt are almost universal. Our sense of reality and purpose was once drawn from the various groups to which we belonged. These entities are now fading, losing their absoluteness, becoming relative. The notion 'global' has so far really only entered into economic life. For it to enter cultural realms we must begin to grasp mankind itself as a great organism, extending over vast ages from its origin into a still distant future. This was the vision of Auguste Comte, the vision Hélan Jaworski developed as the Geon, a living earth with the human being as its brain and thinking, the animals as its feelings, the vegetable kingdom as its life, and the rocks and mountains as its bones. More recently, James Lovelock has been trying to introduce the idea and reality of the living earth, under the name Gaia, into modern science.

This concept of mankind as a whole organism can and must become the content of each individual and will need to be reborn and experienced out of the *free will* of individuals. There are men and women in the world who are 'coming of age' in so far as they are taking personal responsibility as individuals. For others the challenge is extending to the spiritualizing of consciousness in order to integrate hitherto undeveloped parts of the soul, a sort of 'menopausal crisis'. A challenge like this would be answered if each individual could discover that the content of the unconscious is *everyone else*—not only those around us today, but the whole of ancient mankind and future mankind as well. As a human being we are very much a part of the whole human organism, even though the realization of this by the whole of mankind may take millennia to achieve. Our 'unconscious' is only called so because it is not accessible to our intellectual consciousness. It was accessible to the ancient clairvoyant consciousness of earlier cultures and it must in the future become conscious again, as Steiner has indicated, on the levels of living Imagination, Inspiration and Intuition, as these are developed. The abyss that has opened between this world and the spiritual world, between our conscious and unconscious experience, must be bridged. Jung was aware of this abyss and Goethe, somewhat earlier, portrayed the building of such a bridge in his fairy-tale *The Green Snake and the Beautiful Lily*. Individual physicians will have to meet these problems and solve them if medicine is to become a healthy rather than a diseased activity.

Increasing specialization in all walks of life, as well as in medicine, is requiring the development of teams of specialists working together. Here we have a wonderful opportunity to develop social awareness also to a new level. It is common experience today that human problems such as ambition, jealousy and dislikes of various kinds arise in such teamworking and can cause trouble. Pragmatic diplomacy, tact and hypocrisy have been useful and necessary to cope with such situations in the past, but to tackle the problems seriously we need to take a further step. This step will show us that, in any circle of human individuals, when one becomes the problem, or the 'black sheep', it is because all the others are projecting the same human failing that they are harbouring unconsciously in themselves. As the American psychologist Trigant Burrow demonstrated in his book *The Social Basis of Consciousness*, it is the conscious integration of this human failing by the others in themselves that relieves the black sheep, and he is automatically reintegrated in the group. Then the process moves on and, in all likelihood, other problems will surface from unconscious depths. In this way, little by little, we grow beyond the search for objective truth, the dogmatic or infallible truth. Truth is ever moving and developing, it is intrasubjective (i.e., it must arise out of the mutual effort and agreement of all human beings) rather than objective. Our wish to settle for a final truth, which would automatically exclude all others, has been more at home in the past when we recognized partial truths valid for a special geographical area or within a special time period. We seek today the pan-human truth. Dostoevsky proclaimed, 'All men are responsible to all for all.' In the legacy of truths from our human past is contained the affirmation that one man realized in himself the archetype of the whole of mankind. All new truths have to be first realized in one man and the experience of the pan-human truth had first to be realized in one heroic soul. From this stems the possibility for all of us to aim at this perfection, this fulfilment of our human nature. Evolution originated in unconscious unity, developed into individual consciousness and must aim at consciously achieved unity in the future.

The physicians of the future will have to move in these directions or else they will be powerless against ever-increasing soul disorders and new and ever more devastating organically manifesting plagues, epidemics and diseases. We must, in the cause of spirituality or wholeness, be brought to a social awareness of the whole of mankind—past, present and future—and begin to see that all the various categories, associations and even age groups of human beings are, in fact, the organs and supportive functions of the organism of Whole Mankind. Mankind is an organic unity of diverse functions and never was, nor ever will be, merely an undifferentiated entity.

15. Conclusion

We cannot solve the riddles surrounding illness on the ground of natural science alone. Disease processes are as much natural processes as are processes of so-called health. We can even say that they both lead to death. As soon as we prefer health to disease we are introducing value judgements, subjective choice rather than objective observation. In mathematics we are able to reach a shareable truth, but in the realm of values we all dispute. As the saying goes, 'About taste there is no disputing', and Nietzsche's comment in response was, 'There is seldom dispute about anything else.' Up to the present, nobody's judgement about good and evil, about beauty and ugliness, about truth and falsehood is agreed except in the very abstract sphere of mathematics and even there, in higher mathematics, dispute continues. We have also to observe that what is good at one time may be bad at another and so on. So what *is* the truth about illness?

In these ponderings I have tried to indicate directions in which one might find some orientation in all the confusion surrounding problems of disease and healing. What is the meaning of illness? Can we give it meaning? Was Paracelsus on a right track when he regarded illness as opportunity for progress towards salvation or fulfilment?

Mankind has changed over the ages and is, in different parts of the world, differently constituted. Is there an ideal of the universally human—a synthesis of all the ideals of different epochs, races, sexes, religions? In our consciousnesses we are all only partially human; our unconscious selves complete us, for the totality of the rest of humanity is in our unconscious. C.G. Jung showed how the past of all our human evolution and deeds is also in our collective unconscious. All the ancient wisdoms and sciences of our ancestors are still there in our unconscious, but if we attempt to restore them to the light of consciousness we meet certain problems.

Such wisdom of the ancients has come down to us in what is today known as occultism, but the mere mention of this word is enough to provoke violent antagonism in both scientists and churchmen. Yet the ideal of the universally human must also include this memory or legacy from our own past, mostly concealed beneath the threshold of consciousness. This realm of unconscious reality was approachable in ancient times for a dreamlike clairvoyance, but it has since been progressively lost or partly incorporated into traditional theology, accessible now only to faith and not to reason. So arose the schism between what must be accepted by faith alone and what can be reached by thinking. The great Russian philosopher Vladimir Soloviev, however, standing at the pinnacle of European philosophy, was able to show that the mysteries of faith were now accessible to the highest developments of philosophic thought.

Ancient wisdom had been bestowed as a gift to the natural clairvoyance of the time and depended upon the suppression of individuality (which was considered to be illusion). Gradually individuality (and with it moral responsibility) matured and with the coming of Christ reached a point of absolute significance. It has been one of the most important achievements and contributions of Rudolf Steiner to have shown a path to the rebirth of ancient wisdom without compromising our modern wide-awake consciousness or the freedom and responsibility of the individual. The objective and conscious stance towards the outer world achieved by natural science can now be carried over into an awakened consciousness of the spiritual worlds.

For a long time the reality of the spiritual world has been fading for us into a vague, empty abstraction. For Plato the spiritual world or world of Ideas *was* the reality and our world of the senses mere shadows cast on a wall. He stood at the end of the old oriental vision and wisdom, and at the threshold of the dawning occidental science and philosophy. He still had the perception of the pre-existence of the human soul and of reincarnation, which was already lost to his pupil Aristotle. As Steiner has pointed out and emphasized, this loss has led to modern people identifying themselves solely with their hereditary make-up, their DNA. Their uniqueness, their selfhood is thus limited to a particular physical determination confined within the iron law of destiny. To this one-sidedness of the scientific conception Steiner affirmed the other side and indicated the descent of the spiritual individuality from the spiritual cosmos and its uniting with the embryo soon after conception. He was also able to describe the path of this individuality from death to a rebirth. We belong not only to the world of destiny and determinism but also to the world of providence. It is possible for each one of us, in our individual selves, to exercise freedom in choosing the 'possible' of providence rather than the 'necessity' of destiny. It is in this way that meaning can be restored to our lives, and then it will not be just the individual on their personal mystical path but the whole social organism we call mankind that will be enabled to reach its goal.

The intellectual development of recent centuries may have lost us the sense of spiritual worlds, but we have gained as individuals the possibility of freedom. However, this brings with it feelings of isolation and utmost doubt. The increasing separation of our thoughts, feelings and will is crying out for the individuality, the 'I', the ego, to take charge. Our thinking needs to rise out of convention and into our own individually achieved thoughts, and our feelings must develop beyond mere bodily likes and dislikes towards the higher realm of feeling achieved by great artists in their greatest art. Further, our deeds need to become activated by the highest moral ideals and ultimately by Love itself.

It is not surprising that, faced with this challenge, our egos collapse. The symptoms of this are around us in allergic diseases, collapse of the immune system, diabetes, and in the manifestation of evil on an unprecedented scale.

Our egos would gain new confidence if a perception of the dualities of illness were to be cultivated. Health is not a state in itself but the constantly moving healing, or rebalancing, between polar opposite tendencies to disease, and it is the ego that must learn to hold the balance. The idea of healing must be restored to medicine rather than the idea of eliminating various disease entities.

Today there is much talk of holism; mostly it is the idea of a put-together jigsaw picture. We are now able, in coming to the experience of our selves as realities, to begin to rediscover the world of wholes. Wholes are beings, not just bits or pieces of our materially perceptible experience. In this world, the only wholes or spiritual beings commonly known to us are human individuals. The spiritual world is the realm of an almost infinite number of spiritual beings who exist in their consciousnesses but have not physical bodies as we have between birth and death. If we learn to think and then to experience this living world of spiritual beings, our egos will gather courage for the tasks ahead; among such reborn egos new communities would arise based on the recognition and love of other individualities, unique beings, as real as my self.

Bibliography

Adams, G., *Physical and Ethereal Spaces*, Rudolf Steiner Press, London 1965

Adams, G., & Whicher, O., *The Plant between Sun and Earth* (2nd ed.), Rudolf Steiner Press, London 1980

Adams, G., & Whicher, O., *The Living Plant*, Goethean Science Foundation 1949

Adams, G., 'Potentization and the Peripheral Forces of Nature', in *British Homoeopathic Journal*, October 1961

Adler, Alfred, *What Life Should Mean To You*, George Allen & Unwin 1932

Adler, Alfred, *Understanding Human Nature*, George Allen & Unwin 1928

Arber, Agnes, *Goethe's Botany*, Chronica Botanica Co., Waltham, MA 1946

Arber, Agnes, *Natural Philosphy of Plant Form*, Cambridge University Press 1950

Arber, Agnes, *The Manifold and the One*, John Murray 1957

Bahnson, C.B. & M.B., 'Cancer as an Alternative to Psychosis', in *Psychosomatic Aspects of Neoplastic Disease*, Pitman Medical Publishing Co. 1964

Barfield, Owen, 'Historical Perspectives in the Development of Science' in Vol. I of *Towards a Man-centred Medical Science*, eds Karl E. Schaefer, Herbert Hensel and Ronald Brady, Futura Publishing Co., New York 1977

Barfield, Owen, *Saving the Appearances—A Study in Idolatry*, Wesleyan University Press, CT 1965

Bergson, Henri, *Matter and Memory*, George Allen 1913

Bergson, Henri, *Creative Evolution*, Macmillan & Co. 1928

Bergson, Henri, *Time and Free Will*, George Allen & Unwin 1910, 6th impression 1950

Bernard, H.M., *Some Neglected Factors in Evolution*, G.P. Putnam's Sons 1911

Bhagavan Das, *The Science of Social Organization*, 3 vols, Theosophical Publishing House, Adyar 1932, 1935, 1948

Bhagavan Das, *The Science of the Emotions*, Theosophical Publishing House, Adyar 1953

Bjerre, Paul, *Death and Renewal*, Williams & Norgate 1929

Booth, G., 'Cancer and Humanism. Psychosomatic Aspects of Evolution', in *Psychosomatic Aspects of Neoplastic Disease*, Pitman Medical Publishing Co. 1964

Bortoft, H., *Goethe's Scientific Consciousness*, Institute for Cultural Research 1986

Bott, Victor, *Anthroposophical Medicine*, Rudolf Steiner Press 1978

Branfield, Wilfred, *Continuous Creation. A Biological Concept of the Nature of Matter*, Routledge & Kegan Paul, London 1950

Burke, J. Butler, *The Origin of Life*, Chapman & Hall 1906

Burke, J. Butler, *The Emergence of Life*, Oxford University Press 1931

Burrow, T., *The Social Basis of Consciousness*, Kegan Paul 1927

Burrow, T., *The Structure of Insanity*, Kegan Paul 1932

Butler, Samuel, *Unconscious Memory*, A.C. Fifield 1920 (1st ed. 1880)

Butterfield, H., 'Renaissance Art and Modern Science', in *Origins of Scientific Revolution*, Longman 1964

Carrel, Alexis, *Man the Unknown*, Hamish Hamilton 1935

Castiglioni, A., *A History of Medicine*, Alfred Knopf 1941

Chamberlain, H.S., *Immanuel Kant*, 2 vols, Bodley Head 1914

Chambers, R., *Vestiges of the Natural History of Creation*, John Churchill, London 1844

Chauvois, L., *William Harvey*, Hutchinson Medical Publications 1957

Cloos, W., *The Living Earth*, Lanthorn Press 1978

Crombie, A.C., *Augustine to Galileo*, Heineman 1952

Dale-Green, P., *Dog*, Rupert Hart-Davies, London 1966

Eddington, A.S., *The Nature of the Physical World*, Cambridge University Press 1928

Eddington, A.S., *Philosophy of Physical Science*, Cambridge University Press 1928

Eddington, A.S., *New Pathways in Science*, Cambridge University Press 1928

Eiseley, L., *Darwin's Century*, Victor Gollancz 1959

Ellenberger, H.F., *The Discovery of the Unconscious*, Allen Lane, Penguin Press 1970

Fabre d'Olivet, *Hermeneutic Interpretation of the Origin of the Social State in Man*, G.P. Putnam's Sons 1915

Faithfull, T.J., *Plato and the New Psychology*, John Bale Sons & Danielsson 1928

Faithfull, T.J., *Psychological Foundations*, John Bale Sons & Danielsson 1933

Ferenczi, Sandor, 'Thalassa, a Theory of Genitality', in *Psychoanalytic Quarterly*, New York 1938

Ford, Norman M., *When Did I Begin?* Cambridge University Press 1988

Gaskell, W.H., *The Origin of Vertebrates*, Longman Green & Co. 1908

Geikie-Cobb, I., *The Glands of Destiny*, Heinemann 1947

Gould, S.J., *Ontogeny and Phylogeny*, Harvard University Press, Cambridge, MA 1977

Grant Watson, E., *The Mystery of Physical Life*, Abelard Schuman 1964

Glöckler, M., *Medicine at the Threshold of a New Consciousness*, Temple Lodge, London 1997

Groddeck, G., *The Unknown Self*, C.W. Daniel & Co. 1929

Groddeck, G., *Exploring the Unconscious*, C.W. Daniel & Co. 1934

Groddeck, G., *The Book of the It*, Vision Press Ltd. 1950

Groddeck, G., *The World of Man*, C.W. Daniel & Co. 1934

Grohmann, G., *The Plant*, Vol. 1, Rudolf Steiner Press, London 1974

Grohmann, G., *The Plant*, Vol. 2, Biodynamic Farming & Gardening Association 1989

Guirdham, Arthur, *A Theory of Disease*, George Allen & Unwin 1957

Hauschke, R., *The Nature of Substance*, Vincent Stuart 1966

Hiebel, F., *The Gospel of Hellas*, Anthroposophic Press, NY 1949

Illich, I., *Medical Nemesis*, Marion Boyars 1974

Illich, I., *Limits to Medicine*, Marion Boyars 1975

Inglis, Brian, *Revolution in Medicine*, Hutchinson & Co. 1958

Jaworski, H., *Les Étapes de l'histoire*, Maloine et Fils, Paris 1926

Jaworski, H., *Pourquoi la Mort*, J. Oliver, Paris 1926

Jaworski, H., *Après Darwin (l'arbre biologique)*, J.B. Baillière et Fils, Paris 1933

Jaworski, H., *La Decouverte du Monde*, Albin Michel, Paris 1928

Jaworski, H., *La Géon ou la Terre Vivante*, Gallimard, Paris 1928

Jung, C.G., *Modern Man in Search of a Soul*, Kegan Paul 1933

Jung, C.G., *Psychological Types*, Kegan Paul 1923

Jung, C.G., *Two Essays on Analytical Psychology*, Baillière, Tindall & Cox 1928

Jung, C.G., *The Undiscovered Self*, Routledge & Kegan Paul 1958

Kerenyi, K., *The Gods of the Greeks*, Thames & Hudson 1951

Kerenyi, K., *Asklepios*, Thames & Hudson 1960

Kerenyi, K., *Hermes, Guide of Souls*, Spring Publications 1976

Kerenyi, K., *Prometheus*, Thames & Hudson 1963

König, Karl, 'Meditations on the Endocrine Glands', in *The Golden Blade* 1952

Kropotkin, Prince Peter, *Mutual Aid*, Pelican Books 1939

Künkel, F., *In Search of Maturity*, Charles Scribner & Son, NY 1949

Le Fanu, J., *The Rise and Fall of Modern Medicine*, Abacus 1999

Lehrs, E., *Man or Matter*, Faber & Faber 1958

Leroi R., 'Immunologic Events in the Service of the Maintenance of the Human Organism', in *Mercury*, 5, 1981, Spring Valley, NY

Loye, D., *Darwin's Lost Theory of Love*, Excell Press 2000, ISBN 0-595-00131-9

McNeill, W.H., *Plagues and Peoples*, Penguin Books 1977

Mitrinovic, D., *Certainly Future. Selected Writings by Dimitrije Mitrinovic*, East European Monographs, Boulder, CO 1987

Mitrinovic, D., Lectures 1926–1950, J.B. Priestley Library, University of Bradford

Nietzsche, F., *The Birth of Tragedy*, Allen & Unwin 1909

Oken, L., *Elements of Physiophilosophy*, Ray Soc. 1847 (1st German ed. 1810)

Otto, W.F., *The Homeric Gods*, Thames & Hudson 1954

Pagel, W., *The Religious and Philosophical Aspects of Van Helmont's Science and Medicine*, John Hopkins Press 1944

Phillips, E.D., *Greek Medicine*, Thames & Hudson 1973

Poppelbaum, H., *Man and Animal*, Anthroposophical Publishing Co. 1931

Poppelbaum, H., *A New Zoology*, Philosophic Anthroposophic Press 1961

Poppelbaum, H., *A New Light on Heredity and Evolution*, St George Publications, Spring Valley, NY 1977

Portman, A., 'Goethe. The Concept of Metamorphosis', in *Goethe & the Sciences, a Reappraisal*, D. Reidel Publishing Co. 1997

Raven, C.E., *Science, Medicine and Morals*, Hodder & Stoughton 1959

Ripley, W.Z., *The Races of Europe*, Kegan Paul, Trench Trubner 1899

Roszak, Theodore, *The Gendered Atom*, Green Books, Totnes 2000

Sainsbury, G., *The Theory of Polarity*, G.P. Putnam's Sons 1927

Sarton, G., *Ancient Science and Modern Civilization*, Edward Arnold, London 1954

Schaefer, K., *Toward a Man Centred Medical Science*, 3 vols, Futura Publishing Co. 1977

Schrodinger, E., *What is Life?* Doubleday, Garden City, NY 1956

Sherrington, C., *Man on His Nature*, Cambridge University Press 1940

Sigerist, H., *Great Doctors*, George Allen & Unwin 1933

Singer, C., 'How Medicine Became Anatomical', in *British Medical Journal*, 25 December 1954 (Lloyd Roberts' Lecture 1954)

Singer, C., *The Discovery of the Circulation of the Blood*, G. Bell & Sons 1922

Soloviev, V.S., *Anthology*, S.C.M. Press, London 1950

Steiner, R., *Anthroposophical Approach to Medicine*, Anthroposophical Publishing Co., London 1928

Steiner, R., *Goethe, the Scientist*, Anthroposophic Press, New York 1950

Steiner, R., *Pastoral Medicine*, Anthroposophic Press, New York 1987

Steiner, R., *Spiritual Science and Medicine*, Rudolf Steiner Publishing Co., London 1948

Steiner, R., *Spiritual Science and the Art of Healing*, Anthroposophical Publishing Co., London 1950

Steiner, R., *Study of Man*, Rudolf Steiner Publishing Co., London 1947

Steiner, R., *The Universal Human*, Anthroposophic Press, New York 1990

Steiner, R., & Wegman, I., *Fundamentals of Therapy*, Rudolf Steiner Press, London 1967

Stekel, W., *The Beloved Ego*, Kegan Paul, Trench Trubner & Co. 1921

Stirling, J.H., *Darwinism, Workmen and Work*, T. & T. Clark, Edinburgh 1894

Stirner, Max, *The Ego and His Own*, A.C. Fifield, London 1915

Storr, Anthony, 'The Enigma of Music', in *Proceedings of the Royal Society of Medicine*, Vol. 92, January 1999

Thompson, D'Arcy W., *Growth and Form*, Cambridge University Press 1948

Upward, Allen, *The New Word*, Mitchell Kennerley, NY 1910

von Hartmann, E., *The Philosophy of the Unconscious*, 3 vols, Trübner & Co. 1884

Waddington, C.H., *The Nature of Life*, George Allen & Unwin 1961

Wehr, G., *Jung and Steiner*, Anthroposophic Press, New York 2002

Weihs, T.J., *Embryogenesis in Myth and Science*, Floris Books, Edinburgh 1986

Weinniger, O., *Sex and Character*, W. Heinemann, London

Welburn, Andrew, *The Beginnings of Christianity*, Floris Books 1991

Wood Jones, F., *Arboreal Man*, Arnold 1916

Worcester, John, *Physiological Correspondencies*, Boston New Church
    Union 1931
Wilkinson, James Garth, *The Human Body and its Connection with
    Man*, The New Church Press, London 1918